Developing Your Prescribing Skills

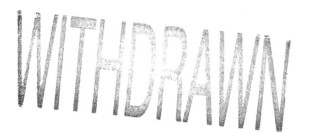

Developing Your Prescribing Skills

Edited by

Trudy Thomas

MRPharmS, GPhC, MSc, BSc
Head of Clinical and Professional
Practice/Taught Postgraduate Programmes Lead
Medway School of Pharmacy
Universities of Greenwich and Kent, UK

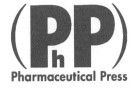

London • Chicago **Pharmaceutical Press**

Published by Pharmaceutical Press

1 Lambeth High Street, London SE1 7JN, UK
1559 St. Paul Avenue, Gurnee, IL 60031, USA

© Pharmaceutical Press 2011

(**P.P**) is a trade mark of Pharmaceutical Press

Pharmaceutical Press is the publishing division of
the Royal Pharmaceutical Society

First published 2011

Typeset by Thomson Digital, Noida, India
Printed in Great Britain by TJ International, Padstow, Cornwall

ISBN 978 0 85369 881 4

A catalogue record for this book is available from the British Library.

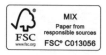

Dedication

I would like to dedicate this book to my family: children Alastair and Kezia and husband Peter, and parents Glenis and Eric. You have all supported me in doing yet one more scary and daft thing in the name of forwarding my career. Thanks for your patience and humour throughout. Also, a huge thanks to colleague and great friend Linda Dodds, who has always believed in me. Finally, a big 'bless you' to all the contributors who bravely came on this big adventure with me.

Contents

Preface

I am a pharmacist with a background in community practice. Indeed, I still practice once a month. Since 1998 I have been lecturing to non-medical prescribers about many aspects of prescribing. I have also worked as a prescribing adviser for a surprising number of Primary Care Trusts (PCTs) over the years, so have worked very closely with prescribers. I have been running the non-medical prescribing programme at the Medway School of Pharmacy since 2004. This programme includes students who are nurses, pharmacists and allied health professionals. Prescribing is dear to my heart.

Why am I editing this book? I have a very clear vision of what it is that prescribers need to think about when prescribing. This is probably very arrogant as I am not a prescriber myself. I love to watch people on our prescribing programme as they develop into prescribers. It is a privilege and pleasure to be part of that change. In this book I am aiming to condense into written form the essence of the learning that our prescribing students go through, with some of the 'spirit' of our programme.

This is why many of the contributors to this book are ex-students or people who teach on the programme. My brief to them has been 'if you could sit down with someone just about to start their prescribing career, what pearls of wisdom would you like to pass on? What are the top tips that you have learned? What mistakes have you made that they should avoid?' This is at the core of this book: the combined experience of 250 years of prescribing – I hope you enjoy it and your prescribing practice.

Trudy Thomas
March 2010

About the editor

Trudy Thomas MSc, BSc, MRPharmS qualified as a pharmacist in 1988. For the next 14 years, she combined community pharmacy work with training and teaching and being a mum. She worked initially for the Centre for Pharmacy Postgraduate Education and the National Pharmaceutical Association, as well as a number of Kent-based Primary Care Organisations, as a prescribing adviser. She joined the Medway School of Pharmacy in 2004, as a clinical lecturer and is now joint Head of Clinical and Professional Practice and Director of Taught Postgraduate Studies. She has been the pharmacist programme lead for the School's Postgraduate Certificate in Independent and Supplementary Prescribing for 6 years.

Trudy's research interests are mainly to do with prescribing and physical activity. In 2008 she started a part-time PhD investigating whether community pharmacists can use behaviour change counselling to increase the amount of physical activity undertaken by people with mild to moderate depression.

Trudy is a keen runner and cyclist.

Contributors

Angela Black MSc, GradDipPhys, MCSP

Angela qualified as physiotherapist in 1986 and immediately started work at Medway Hospital. After completing general rotations she transferred into the community paediatric physiotherapy team. This team has expanded over the years and is now a large multidisciplinary team which consists of members from five allied health professions and includes specialist nurses. Her role in the team is as the principal physiotherapist, specialising in the area of neurodisability. In this role, she qualified as a supplementary prescriber from Medway School of Pharmacy in 2006. Since then she has been able to integrate her prescribing practice to enhance the provision of therapy intervention for children who present with spasticity.

Jane Colbert RGN, BSc(Hons), NP, Dip(RCN).NMP

Jane is currently nurse prescribing lead for the Postgraduate Certificate in Independent and Supplementary Prescribing at the Medway School of Pharmacy. Her experience of working both as a nurse practitioner in the community and latterly as a nurse prescriber led to an interest and natural inclination towards education. The evolutionary processes inherent in both preparation and learning to become a prescriber are of particular interest, with consultation skills being the main focus.

Stuart Gill-Banham BSc(Hons), MRPharmS

Stuart is a pharmacist with many years' experience working in mental health care teams. This has covered adult, elderly, forensic, learning disabilities and children's services. From 2003 to 2007 he was the first elected registrar of the College of Mental Health Pharmacists. Stuart continues to be involved in national courses run by the CMHP that aim to develop pharmacists working within psychiatry. At the Medway School of Pharmacy Stuart leads the teaching in psychiatry and neurology at both undergraduate and postgraduate level. He has been involved with the School's non-medical prescribing programme since its inception in 2004 and has guided many students through the course who have gone on to prescribe in a range of mental health and substance misuse settings.

Michael Jenkinson BSc(Hons), MBChB, FRCP

Michael is a consultant physician practising since 1992 in Margate in Kent. While training he had experience in clinical pharmacology at the University of Otago, Dunedin, New Zealand, in Adelaide, Australia and at the New Cross National Poisons Unit, London. He is presently lead clinician drugs and therapeutics for the East Kent Hospitals University Foundation Trust. He is also a member of the South East Coast Policy Recommendation Committee and the High Cost Drugs Group, The NHS Information Centre for Health & Social Care. He contributes to an educational wiki orientated towards doctors called GANFYD (http://www.ganfyd.org), which has about a 50% year on year growth in hits.

Deborah Jenner RGN, DipHE, BSc(Hons), PgCert (Indep. Presc.)

Deborah qualified as a registered nurse in 1981 and worked as a staff nurse in general surgery until she had her children, when she had a career break. She began hospice nursing in 1993 and after a period of out-of-hours community nursing, began her degree in palliative care nursing and secured a position as a community-based clinical nurse specialist (CNS) in palliative care in 2002. After 3 years she moved into her current role as CNS in palliative care in an acute hospital team. Wishing to develop this role, she undertook and completed her Postgraduate Certificate in Independent Nurse Prescribing in 2008. Deborah finds this to be a satisfying and invaluable qualification and skill, enabling her to deliver prompt and timely treatment to patients using her knowledge and experience to inform practice.

Derek Meadows BSc, PgCert (Indep. Presc.), MRPharmS

Derek is a pharmacist independent prescriber. He initially qualified as a supplementary prescriber at Christchurch College, Canterbury and practised in that role for 2 years, building up his prescribing experience. He completed the Independent Prescribing module at the Medway School of Pharmacy, and has prescribed continuously in his role as pharmacist within the Charing Medical Practice in Kent, supported and mentored by the general practitioner partners.

Hilary Pinnock MB, ChB, MRCGP, MD

Hilary is a general practitioner at the Whitstable Medical Practice, Kent. She is also a senior clinical research fellow with the Allergy and Respiratory Research Group, Centre for Population Health Sciences: GP Section, University of Edinburgh, where she is supported by a Primary Care Research Career Award from the Chief Scientist Office of the Scottish Government.

Her research interests include the delivery of care within the 'real-life' primary care setting, including telephone reviews for asthma, and telehealth for monitoring respiratory disease, the palliative care needs of people with chronic obstructive pulmonary disease (COPD) and the role of GPs with a special interest. She is co-lead of the Education Subgroup of the International Primary Care Respiratory Group, and is actively involved in the education programme of the Primary Care Respiratory Society UK. She chairs the self-management evidence review group of the BTS-SIGN asthma guideline, and contributed to the COPD National Strategy.

Greg Rogers MB, ChB, FRCGP, MSc [epileptology], DRCOG

Greg is a general practitioner in Margate and the East Kent clinical lead special interest in epilepsy. He has been involved in epilepsy care for many years and has established links to the epilepsy charities Epilepsy Action and Epilepsy Bereaved in the capacity of clinical adviser. He has also worked for the Department of Health, being one of the national advisers for the 18-week Blackout Pathway; he also sits on the NICE Guideline Review Panel and worked on three guideline development groups (Transient Loss of Consciousness, Epilepsy Update and Non-invasive Ventilation for Motor Neurone Disease).

His interest in community service provision and redesign has led him to develop closer links to the work of pharmacists and he is a firm advocate for embedding the skills of pharmacists more deeply into the primary healthcare team. In his spare time he keeps some rather spoiled chickens!

Debbie Smart

Debbie qualified as an RGN at Tunbridge Wells School of Nursing. Following her marriage, she moved to Yorkshire where she worked at Castle Hill Hospital in Cottingham as a staff nurse on a thoracic medicine unit for 6 years, progressing to acting sister. She moved back to Kent into general practice and had her two children. Over the next few years she undertook qualifications in coronary heart disease, diabetes, women's health, family planning and minor illness. She completed her non-medical prescribing in 2008 and is now a lead nurse at St Mary's Medical Centre in Kent.

Elizabeth Worthing BPharm (Wales), MSc (Clin. Pharm.), ATAP, MRPharmS

Liz is a UK trained pharmacist with hospital and teaching experience in Britain, East Africa, Papua New Guinea, Australia and Oman. After registration she worked briefly at Great Ormond Street Hospital for Children, and later developed her paediatric specialisation and teaching experience with medical and pharmacy students in Muscat. She is currently based at Medway Maritime Hospital with 50% secondment to Medway School of Pharmacy. She has a special interest in asthma and provides paediatric input into the Independent and Supplementary Prescribing Course.

Abbreviations

ADR	adverse drug reaction
ALP	alanine aminotransferase
AST	aspartate aminotransferase
BMI	body mass index
BNF	*British National Formulary*
CABG	coronary artery bypass graft
CRP	C-reactive protein
CSCI	continuous subcutaneous infusion
DOB	date of birth
ECG	electrocardiogram
EEG	electroencephalogram
eGFR	estimated glomerular filtration rate
FBC	full blood count
GGT	gamma-glutamyltransferase
GI	gastrointestinal
GP	general practitioner
GSL	General Sales List
HDL	high-density lipoprotein
Hb	haemoglobin
HbA1c	haemoglobin A1C
HR	heart rate
IFCC	International Federation of Clinical Chemistry
INR	International Normalised Ratio
LDL	low-density lipoprotein
MRI	magnetic resonance imaging
NSTEMI	non-ST elevation myocardial infarction
OTC	over the counter
P	Pharmacy Only Medicines
PCO	Primary Care Organisation
PCT	Primary Care Trust
PEFR	peak expiratory flow rate
pMDI	pressurised metered dose inhaler
POM	Prescription Only Medicines

SR	sustained release
SVD	spontaneous vaginal delivery
TC	total cholesterol
TIA	transient ischaemic attack
TURP	transurethral resection of the prostate
U&Es	urea and electrolytes

1

Introduction to prescribing and this book

Trudy Thomas

Historical origins of prescribing

The Oxford English Dictionary defines prescribing as 'the ordering of a use of a medicine'. It comes from the Latin *pre*, meaning 'before' and *scribo*, meaning 'to write', so is an order written before a medicine can be prepared.

It is possible that the first prescriptions were written on clay tablets by healers in Babylon around 2600 BC, with the symptoms of disease, as well as the prescription and directions for the compounding of plants and herbs and prayers to the gods being recorded (Washington State University, 1995). Records from 1550 BC, the 'Papyrus Ebers', a collection of 800 prescriptions, mention 700 different drugs and are evidence that prescribing and dispensing were firmly established in Ancient Egypt.

The original Hippocratic Oath from the fourth century BC is said to include the sentence 'I will prescribe regimens for the good of my patients according to my ability and my judgment, and never do harm to anyone.' A suitable aspiration for all prescribers, one might hope, although this wording has been replaced in more modern versions by something akin to 'I will follow that method of treatment which according to my ability and judgment, I consider for the benefit of my patient and abstain from whatever is harmful or mischievous'.

The origins of the symbol 'Rx' are unclear. It is possible that it is a shortening of the Latin word *recipere* meaning 'take back' and is in fact a command to the pharmacist from the prescriber to 'take these ingredients and make this medicine', rather than an instruction to the patient to take the medicine.

Prescribing today

However ancient its origins, the prescribing of medicines is very much part of the prevention and management of disease in the modern world. Once purely the domain of the physician, changes in legislation in the United Kingdom that started in the late 1980s have finally seen the legal right to prescribe conferred to other healthcare professionals (non-medical prescribers), including nurses, pharmacists and certain allied health professionals. These professionals undertake additional training to qualify as: independent and supplementary prescribers (a dual qualification) in the case of nurses and pharmacists; supplementary prescribers in the case of physiotherapists, podiatrists and radiographers; and as independent prescribers (from a limited formulary) in the case of optometrists. The introduction of non-medical prescribing has been a gradual process and is still evolving. At the time of writing, legislation that extends non-medical prescribers' ability to prescribe controlled drugs is still to be finalised. It is possible that other professional groups will also prescribe in the future (Department of Health, 2010).

If you write a prescription for a medicine in the UK (or sign one written by someone else) you are legally and clinically responsible for the consequences. All prescribers should be familiar with the Medicines Act 1968 and the Misuse of Drugs Act 1971. If you make a prescribing error you could be in breach of one (or both) of these Acts and could be liable to prosecution under the Act.

Concerns about litigation, as well as advances in technology, among other factors, have led to a reduction in the compounding of medicines (extemporaneous dispensing) in the pharmacy. Medicines that are prescribed and made in this way have no licence (authorisation) and so present a greater risk to both patient (and prescriber). In the 12 months to January 2009 there were around 10 000 items endorsed by community pharmacists as 'extemporaneously dispensed' (NHS Prescription Services Information systems, 2009). This represents a tiny fraction of the total items prescribed, but does indicate that the prescribing and preparation of these unlicensed medicines is still required. In the hospital sector, and especially in paediatric medicine, the manufacture of unlicensed medicines is much greater (one study in 2004 suggested the average number of products extemporaneously prepared was 1.5 per paediatric department per day; Yeung *et al.*, 2004).

The reduction in extemporaneously prepared items, the advent of evidence-based medicine and financial constraints appear to have constricted the range of medicines prescribed. Working in the pharmacy now, one is conscious of a much more 'formulaic' approach to the management of disease. By the time the person with type 2 diabetes has arrived at the dispensing counter, the ramipril 10 mg, simvastatin 40 mg and aspirin 75 mg are already on the bench and the hand is hovering over the two strengths of metformin. Quite right and proper one might say, but undoubtedly others would argue that some of the 'art' of prescribing has been lost.

The prescribing canvas

The idea that prescribing is an art is useful when we consider the skills needed by the prescriber of today. As an artist, every prescriber must consider the canvas on which they will be prescribing. It is seldom blank! When prescribing for a patient with type 2 diabetes, the prescriber will also have to take into consideration this person's blood pressure, weight management and cholesterol. The prescriber may be managing those aspects of the patient's care anyway. However, if this patient also has epilepsy, the prescriber may not be prescribing for that condition, but will have to be mindful of the effects his or her prescribing will have on the management of this person's epilepsy. Many new prescribers will be acutely aware that there may be drug interactions between the diabetes treatment and the antiepileptic agents; however, they also need to consider the effect of the diabetes medication on the epilepsy itself. So, potentially as the prescriber prescribes for the patient's condition this could interfere with another aspect (in this example the epilepsy) and likewise the management of the epilepsy could affect the person's diabetic control.

It doesn't have to be that the two medicines interact in terms of their active ingredients. It is possible that the actions of one medication may adversely affect the other medication because of its formulation. For example, the dry mouth caused by medication with an anticholinergic action may prevent the effective dissolution of sublingual medication, such as GTN tablets.

Of course the 'canvas' also includes the patient themselves. Prescribing will be different for a child or an older person because the pharmacokinetics are altered in different age groups and in patients with different co-morbidities. We touch on this in a number of the chapters that follow and offer some general strategies. One canvas that makes prescribing very challenging is when the patient is pregnant or breastfeeding. We have deliberately not included a chapter in which the patient is pregnant or breastfeeding because this is such a difficult area to discuss and making generalisations is unhelpful. Every patient case is different and the approaches taken by the experts in this book cannot safely be applied wholesale to any other patient, unless they were identical in every aspect to the one described. However, if there is one area where the decision to prescribe must be absolutely tailored to the individual more than any other, it is in the area of prescribing in pregnancy. The consequences of prescribing for a pregnant woman are manifold and the risks must always be weighed against the benefits for that individual. The most important single piece of advice all the experts in this book could offer to any other prescriber, however, is *always* ask about pregnancy. Imagine prescribing a drug for a patient, only to discover that she is pregnant afterwards. The fact that your patient didn't offer the information and you didn't ask would not stand up in a court of law, nor is it likely to appease your conscience if something dreadful were to happen to the unborn child. You must *always* establish if the patient could be pregnant and if there is even the smallest chance, then you must assume that she is. Do not assume that a woman in her 40s or even 50s could not be pregnant. Just because a woman wasn't pregnant last time you saw her, doesn't mean she isn't pregnant the next time!

Safe prescribing

The ultimate aim of any prescriber must be to be safe and effective. A recent report on behalf of the General Medical Council (Dornan *et al.*, 2009) carried out across 19 hospitals in north-west England found that there was an 8.9% prescribing error rate. The study looked specifically at Foundation Year 1 (FY1) doctors who demonstrated an error rate of 8.4%. All grades of doctor (including consultants) and nurses made prescribing errors. The highest error rate was found in Foundation Year 2 (FY2) doctors (10.3%). In most cases the errors were detected by pharmacists in the hospital before they could cause harm. This study was the first to report on prescribing error rates in non-medical prescribers (nurses and pharmacists). These professionals were shown to have a similar error rate to consultants, which was lower than that for the junior doctors. While this might be comforting to supporters of non-medical prescribing, it is not appropriate to say that this is an acceptable error rate. All prescribers must strive to get as close to zero prescribing errors as possible. Every single error that results in harm or distress to a patient is one too many.

The National Patient Safety Agency (NPSA) for England and Wales saw some 86 000 medication incidents reported to its Reporting and Learning System (RLS) in 2007 (NPSA, 2009). This represented 9% of all incidents reported to the RLS (third in volume after patient accidents and incidents with treatments/procedures). The vast majority of reported medication-related incidents resulted in low or no harm to the patient. There were, however, 100 reports of death and severe harm via the RLS in this timeframe.

Medicines administration was associated with 41% of these reports, with prescribing per se attributed to 32%. Incidents involving injectable medicines represented 62% of all reported incidents leading to death or severe harm. The researchers classified the errors into three types, which together represented 71% of all fatal or severe harm errors. These were: (1) unclear or wrong dose or wrong frequency; (2) wrong medicine; and (3) omitted or delayed medicines.

The types of medicines most frequently associated with severe harm included cardiovascular medicines, anti-infective agents, opioids, anti-coagulants and antiplatelet medicines. A number of these also featured in the study by Pirmohamed *et al.* (2001). This work looked at admissions to two hospitals over a six-month period to determine how many were attributable to adverse drug reactions (ADRs). Of the approximately 18 500 patients admitted during the time of the study, 1225 (6.5%) were considered to be related to an ADR. The overall fatality was 0.15%. Most reactions were classified as 'definitely or possibly avoidable'. Medicines most commonly implicated in causing these admissions included aspirin (low dose), diuretics, warfarin and non-steroidal anti-inflammatory drugs (other than aspirin). The main adverse drug reaction found was gastrointestinal bleeding.

The GMC study (Dornan, 2009) mentioned earlier, also looked at the causes of the errors made. Errors were less likely to be due to knowledge deficiencies alone. If a prescriber was aware that they did not know something, they would generally make a conscious decision to look it up, or seek help. (Of course this support may not be available or reliable at the time and the error may still occur.) Errors were shown to occur more often when the person made a 'slip'. This was more likely to happen when the person was familiar with the 'rules' of the task. They knew the 'right' thing to do, or the 'right' way to do something, but for some reason, unintentionally, did not apply the 'rule' in the right way at the right time. It may be that many of these 'rule-based activities' are things we do all the time, almost on automatic. There is little cognitive functioning occurring at the time of the slip. This also explains why people who make medication errors are often unaware of what they have done.

Usually it is a complex set of circumstances that lead to a mistake being made. One might think it is difficult to mitigate against such events; we are, after all, human. Perhaps just being mindful of common mistakes and how they can occur is the prescriber's best defence. Complacency is possibly the prescriber's greatest enemy. In the GMC report the FY2s made more errors than the FY1s.

Effective prescribing

One certain way to be the safest prescriber would be never to prescribe anything. However, to *not* prescribe when one is qualified as a prescriber *is* a prescribing decision and one must always consider the consequences to the patient of not prescribing. The RLS study (NPSA, 2009) classified omission or delay of prescription as an error.

It may be an obvious point, but it is worth remembering that just because you can legally prescribe everything in the *British National Formulary* (BNF) (Joint Formulary Committee, 2010), doesn't mean you are going to. Each prescriber should have an agreed 'scope of prescribing practice' which means he or she can offer a safe and effective service to patients. This 'service' needs to make sense to the people commissioning it. A novice prescriber is unlikely to be able to say 'I'd like to prescribe for people with asthma, but prednisolone has got a lot of nasty side-effects, so I won't write prescriptions for that'.

For some prescribers working in a specialist clinical area the scope of prescribing practice may be quite limited in terms of the medicines they prescribe. Those prescribers will (and should) know those medicines inside-out. They must know the place of each medicine in clinical practice, the evidence base behind it and the pharmacokinetics and dynamics that apply. Prescribers working in more general settings may be required to prescribe a much wider range of medicines. In this case it is not possible to know everything about every medicine in the same depth. The World Health Organization *Guide to Good Prescribing* suggests that each prescriber should be familiar with their personal formulary of medicines (or 'P drugs') (WHO, 2004). The P drugs are the 40–60 medicines that the more generalist prescriber will prescribe routinely. The Guide offers a method by which the prescriber selects his or her P drugs, which includes:

- defining the diagnosis (pathophysiology);
- specifying the therapeutic objective;
- making an inventory of effective medicine groups;
- choosing a group according to criteria (efficacy, safety, suitability and cost); and
- choosing a P drug (and if necessary an alternative) within the group, again considering efficacy, safety, suitability and cost. This also includes consideration of the dosage form and standard dose range and duration of therapy.

The Guide makes the distinction between a P drug and a P treatment. This places pharmacological treatment appropriately with non-pharmacological treatment including general and lifestyle advice. Just because someone is a prescriber, it does not mean that the treatment for every condition is a medicine.

Although it was written some considerable time ago, the WHO Guide offers a sensible approach to scoping one's practice and also suggests a way to consider how as a prescriber one includes new medicines (or not) into one's repertoire. It makes the key point that just because a medicine is new, it doesn't make it any good. On the other hand, being totally cynical and ignoring new products is equally wrong. A dose of healthy scepticism when considering a new product is probably a wise starting point.

Principles of prescribing

Many organisations offer guidance and advice on prescribing. The GMC 'Good practice in prescribing medicines – guidance for doctors' is a good starting point, regardless of your professional background (GMC, 2008). The National Prescribing Centre offers extensive resources and provides essential support for all prescribers. (www.npc.co.uk). For some very practical advice on writing prescriptions, there is nowhere better to go than the front of the BNF (Joint Formulary Committee, 2010), where there is advice entitled 'Guidance on prescribing'. It is surprising how many experienced prescribers don't know it is there!

You will find the prescribing 'security blankets' (i.e. useful guidelines, websites and other resources) used by the prescribers who have contributed to this book at the end of each chapter. You will have your own favourites too, of course. These should be reputable sources, with a known provenance, that are updated regularly. They should not be open websites that can have material contributed by anyone.

Over the course of your career, probably the greatest learning resource will be your colleagues and patients. We have tried to supply some of both for you in this book.

What this book is and isn't

This book is not an evidence-based text book, designed to give you indepth knowledge on any aspect of pharmacology that you may wish to consider. There are many excellent books on the market that will fulfil this need, if facts and figures are what you are after. Indeed many of the chapters list other sources of information and evidence-based references that you might go to if you wish to research further into the subject. Our feeling when writing this book was that what prescribing students want to know isn't something that a conventional text book will tell them. In this book the authors are trying to pass on aspects of their experience in prescribing and to provide some things to think about. The chapters take an unashamedly personal view. In many cases there isn't a right or wrong answer. Sometimes it is the 'least wrong' that is what we have to settle for in real life.

The scenarios enable the authors to look at some key aspects common to prescribing across the board. We do not pretend that we offer the definitive and comprehensive answer. The 'answer' to one patient's problem will be very different from another's and by presenting some common prescribing dilemmas, we hope this will at least raise awareness of things to think about when prescribing. We are not saying 'this is how to prescribe – do it like this' but we are saying 'in this scenario these are the possible pitfalls and these are the things to look out for'.

How to use this book

Each subsequent chapter of this book consists of at least one patient scenario. The scenario is set in the clinical area in which the chapter author is a specialist. The majority of the authors are prescribers; however, those who are not have all worked closely with prescribers and so all have a personal view to offer on aspects of prescribing practice. In a way, the clinical setting of the scenario is less important. It is merely the backdrop to the generic prescribing issues which are the real subject of the chapter. You do not have to be an expert in the clinical topic to appreciate the issues being considered. In Chapter 2, for example, the prescriber (and chapter author) is a pharmacist with expertise in anticoagulation. You may never prescribe anticoagulants in your life, you may never even prescribe 'your' medicines for someone taking anticoagulants. However, the subject of the chapter, accountability and responsibility, is something that is applicable to all prescribers, whatever medications they prescribe and whoever they prescribe them for.

Introduction and learning outcomes

Each chapter starts with a brief introduction to the chapter, the clinical setting and the prescriber who features in the chapter. While the prescriber and the chapter author may have similarities and characteristics in common, there is a fundamental difference in that the prescriber is fictitious. Sometimes the best learning takes place after there has been a problem in practice. We wanted to give our fictitious prescribers the freedom to make mistakes if necessary in the scenario, so we could all learn from their errors.

We want this book to help you in your learning and so we have tried to give it an interactive feel by introducing reflective questions. These will be discussed in a moment. The learning outcomes show you what is covered by the chapter. Looking back at these at the end of the chapter will help you recognise what learning has taken place and also help you identify any further gaps in your learning. You can then refer to the mind map at the end of the chapter, to see which other chapters in the book might help to fill these gaps. You do not have to work through the chapters in numerical order – let your identified learning needs guide your route through.

The patient

We are introduced to the patient 'star' of the scenario in this section. All case studies are based on real patients and some of the little details and red herrings that inevitably come with patients have been left in to try to bring each patient alive on the page. Each patient has a background information sheet. This is a potted medical history, which you will need to refer to when considering the prescribing issues posed by the scenario. In some cases, the scenario is chunked up, so that we might pick up the story again days, months or even years later. This gives our prescriber the chance to build on his or her previous successes or learn from previous mistakes.

Reflective questions

Each scenario poses a number of reflective questions. You can use these to 'test yourself' by looking at these questions and considering what you think are the key points. You might like to jot them down in a notebook, for example. The recording of your reflection can be used as part of the record of your continuing professional development. The thoughts of the author follow on after the reflective questions. You may think of other aspects in relation to these cases. We hope that as a student or new prescriber you will have the opportunity to discuss your thoughts with a more experienced colleague. You could even use the cases as part of a learning set or discussion group. Once you have worked through the reflective questions, in whatever way suits you, you can then look at the suggested responses from the chapter author. The reflective questions usually relate to the generic issues being raised in the scenario, although we do get some clinical details from our experts as well.

Prescribing pitfalls and top tips

These are the do's and don'ts of prescribing as suggested by the chapter author. Some of the points may seem obvious to you, but we find that sometimes the basics get overlooked with prescribing because there are so many other more complex things that need to be thought about.

Mind maps

Each chapter focuses on one subject in detail, but inevitably other aspects of prescribing will be touched upon in the chapter. Each chapter ends with a mind map. The mind map will show you where in the book these topics are covered in more detail and how related subjects fit together.

References, websites and further reading

Each chapter concludes with resources which the author finds useful in their clinical and prescribing practice. The idea was not to produce an exhaustive reference list, but give you some key places to start if you wish to read further on the topic discussed and the clinical condition covered in the chapter.

A note on dates

To avoid the patients ageing with the book, dates have been presented in the form *'n years ago'*. Thus a patient's date of birth might be presented as *1/1/seventy years ago*, or an event as *'MI 3 years ago'*.

References

Department of Health (2010) Allied health professions prescribing and medicines supply mechanisms scoping project report. Available at: www.dh.gov.uk/prod_consum_dh/groups/dh_digitalassets/documents/digitalasset/dh_103949.pdf [Accessed June 2010].

Dornan T, Ashcroft D, Heathfield H, *et al.* (2009) An in depth investigation into causes of prescribing errors by foundation trainees in relation to their medical education. EQUIP study. Available at: www.gmc-uk.org/FINAL_Report_prevalence_and_causes_of_prescribing_errors.pdf_28935150.pdf [Accessed 23 March 2010].

GMC (General Medical Council) (2008) Good practice in prescribing medicines – guidance for doctors. Available at: www.gmc-uk.org/guidance/ethical_guidance/prescriptions_faqs.asp [Accessed 23 March 2010].

Joint Formulary Committee (2010) *BNF: British National Formulary 60.* London: British Medical Association and Royal Pharmaceutical Society of Great Britain.

NHS Prescription Services Information systems (2009) Extemporaneous dispensing, England, February 2004 to January 2009. Available at: www.ppa.org.uk/foidocs/responses/FOI_Request_(447866a).pdf [Accessed 23 March 2010].

NPSA (National Patient Safety Agency) (2009) National Learning Reporting Service. 2009. Safety in doses. Available at: www.nrls.npsa.nhs.uk/resources/patient-safety-topics/medication-safety/?entryid45=61625&p=2 [Accessed 23 March 2010].

Pirmohamed M, James S, Meakin S *et al.* (2001) Adverse drug reactions as cause of admission to hospital: prospective analysis of 18 820 patients. *British Medical Journal* 329(7456): 15–19.

Washington State University (1995) College of Pharmacy. History of pharmacy. Available at: www.pharmacy.wsu.edu/History/history04.html [Accessed 5 January 2010].

WHO (World Health Organization) (2004) Guide to good prescribing. Available at: http://apps.who.int/medicinedocs/pdf/whozip23e/whozip23e.pdf [Accessed 23 March 2010].

Yeung VW, Tuleut CLC, Wong ICK (2004) National study of extemporaneous preparations in English paediatric hospital pharmacies. *Paediatric and Perinatal Drug Therapy* 6: 75–80.

Further reading/websites of interest

Bradley E and Nolan P (2008) *Non-Medical Prescribing: Multidisciplinary perspectives.* Cambridge: Cambridge University Press.

British National Formulary online. http//bnf.org

Brookes D and Smith A (2006) *Non-medical Prescribing in healthcare Practice: a tool kit for students and practitioners.* Basingstoke: Palgrave Macmillan.

Courtney M and Griffiths M (2004) *Independent and Supplementary Prescribing: an essential guide.* Cambridge: Cambridge University Press.

Crichton B (2006) *Fundamentals of Primary Care Prescribing.* London: Royal College of General Practitioners.

Department of Health (2010) The non-medical prescribing programme. http://webarchive.nationalarchives.gov.uk/+/www.dh.gov.uk/en/Healthcare/Medicinespharmacyandindustry/Prescriptions/TheNon-MedicalPrescribingProgramme/index.htm [Accessed June 2010].

Dowell J, Williams B and Snadden D (2007) *Patient Centred Prescribing.* Oxford: Radcliffe Publishing.

Jones O and Gautam N (2003) *The Hands-on Guide to Practical Prescribing.* Oxford: Wiley-Blackwell.

McGavock H (2009) *Pitfalls in Prescribing and How to Avoid Them.* Oxford: Radcliffe Publishing.

National Prescribing Centre. www.npc.co.uk

Waite M, Keenan J (2009) *CPD for Non Medical Prescribers: a practical guide.* Oxford: Wiley-Blackwell.

2

Being accountable for your prescribing

Derek Meadows

Learning outcomes

After completing this chapter you will be able to:

- identify the lines of responsibility and accountability for prescribers;
- discuss what it means to 'prescribe within one's area of competency';
- outline key principles involved in dealing with prescribing errors.

Introduction

This chapter demonstrates that with one lapse of judgement the prescriber can fail to fulfil their obligations to the patient, professional colleagues, commissioning body and themselves. It shows how easy it is for the inexperienced prescriber to be deflected from prescribing safely and effectively. It highlights the importance of remaining focused and not being unduly influenced by the expectations of the patient or professional colleagues, whether real or perceived. The desire to please can lead the unwary prescriber to take unnecessary risks, leaving them exposed to criticism or even litigation.

Prescriber

David Mitchell is the pharmacy superintendant of a community pharmacy located within a general practitioner (GP) surgery. The limited company is wholly owned by the partners in the doctors' practice.

David is responsible for all the professional, ethical, legal and commercial aspects of the business and enjoys a large degree of autonomy in his day-to-day activity. He has recently sought to expand his personal competencies by qualifying as an independent pharmacist prescriber specialising in anticoagulation.

David uses his expertise by running an anticoagulant clinic three afternoons a week at the practice. This is run as a locally enhanced service for the Primary Care Organisation (PCO). There is currently a drive to move this service from secondary care to primary care as demand increases with an ageing population and the desire to make the service more accessible to patients (Department of Health, 2008). David has full access to the GPs' patient records.

Patient background

Graham Rogers is a 53-year-old male self-employed entrepreneur. He lives with his wife and teenage daughter on a smallholding which he purchased for the stabling. His family are keen on horses, and domestic life centres around their hobby. Graham has just purchased a new company installing CCTV cameras. Life at the moment is pretty stressful. He has two ways of winding down at the end of the day. The first is to grab a fork and wheelbarrow and attend to mucking out the stables. This is his only exercise which, like everything else in his life, he does at full speed. Having spent an hour labouring he relaxes with a meal, washed down with a whole bottle of red wine (his second wind-down technique).

Recently he has noticed that he does not have the energy he used to have and has to pace himself to get through his evening's physical work. He will often fall asleep on the sofa when watching the television. He has been on medication for hypertension for two years now and occasionally has to see his GP for treatment for gout, which in his view is a minor inconvenience compared to the benefits he considers he gets from his evening drink.

Taking advantage of his private medical cover, Graham arranges for a private health check-up at a time of his convenience to see if he can get to the bottom of his lack of stamina. The results indicate that he has persistent atrial fibrillation.

The diagnosis is reported back to the patient's GP, who in turn sends Graham to see David to arrange anticoagulation with warfarin. He simultaneously refers him to the cardiologist at the hospital for further investigation.

Summary sheet with background information

Name: Graham Rogers
DOB: 29/5/*fifty-three years ago*
Occupation: Self-employed business entrepreneur

Past medical history

Chicken pox aged 5 years
Immunisation status – all available childhood vaccinations had at
    the appropriate age
Hep A and B and tetanus vaccinations *two years ago*
Hypertension *diagnosed two years ago*
Gout *diagnosed 18 months ago*

Current medication (last dispensed three weeks ago)

Aspirin 75 mg one in the morning
Atenolol 50 mg one in the morning
Nifedipine XL 30 mg one morning and night

Disease monitoring (carried out at private health check one week ago)

BMI: 27
Blood pressure: 157/90 mmHg
Pulse: irregularly irregular, rate 170 bpm
ECG: Shows P wave replaced by rapid oscillations of varying size,
    shape and timing
Thyroid, liver function test, U&Es, full blood count, cholesterol –
    normal
Random blood sugar: 7.9 mmol/L

Social history

Married with teenage daughter
Smokes 15 cigarettes per day
Alcohol: ++
Physical activity: mucks out horses every day

Because of his work commitments, the first time Graham can keep an appointment is Friday 3 March in the afternoon. As he enters the room it is apparent that he is both apprehensive and very low in mood.

> *I've been told I've got to go on warfarin. I know that thins the blood, my doctor told me, so that means I'll be even more tired now! And don't you start nagging me about not taking my blood pressure pills, I get enough of that from my wife and I've just had an earful from the doctor.*

He then adds, 'Can I still go paintballing with my mates on Saturday?'

As part of the comprehensive patient history, David discovers that Graham has uncontrolled hypertension, poor compliance and a high alcohol intake, all increased risk factors for unwanted bleeding in patients taking warfarin. David is not convinced of the benefits of anticoagulation compared to the risks of a potential major bleed. He attempts to contact Graham's doctor to discuss the case, but the GP is not available until Monday. David decides to postpone starting anticoagulation until after the weekend. He recognises that this could result in a week's delay to starting therapy, as Graham is working until the following Friday. However, David discusses this with Graham, who seems unconcerned.

On Monday 6 March, David contacts the GP who is not at all supportive of his actions. The GP points out that National Institute for Health and Clinical Excellence (NICE) guidelines make it quite clear that anticoagulation with warfarin is indicated and that by delaying the start of therapy David has put the patient at risk of stroke unnecessarily for a week. David is now concerned that lack of experience has led him to make a poor clinical decision. He is also mindful of his need to maintain credibility with the doctors' practice both personally and professionally. In an attempt to bring forward the anticoagulation, David telephones the patient. However, Graham still cannot commit to the appointments needed for a conventional loading regimen, which would require him to attend the pharmacy over a period of at least two weeks.

David, now feeling under pressure, negotiates with Graham a fast-loading scheme usually used in hospital known as Fennerty. In this regimen, the patient is given 10 mg of warfarin each day with daily INR (International Normalised Ratio) checks. The dose is reduced as soon as the patient's INR climbs towards the therapeutic target of 2.5, usually by day 3 (Baglin *et al.*, 2005). (A variation of 0.5 either side of this target is considered satisfactory.) Graham likes the 'get stuck in approach', as he calls it, and agrees to call in at 9am sharp to start the regimen before he begins work. However, the first day he can make is Wednesday 8 March. David completes Graham's treatment record card recording the dose of warfarin prescribed. He also gives Graham the National Patient Safety Agency (NPSA) yellow information booklet on anticoagulation (NPSA, 2007), which Graham agrees to read 'when he gets a minute'.

Wednesday arrives and, to David's relief, Graham attends for his appointment. His INR is recorded as 1.1 and David instructs him to take 10 mg of warfarin at 6pm. On Thursday morning, his INR has not changed. David instructs Graham to take another 10 mg that evening. David believes that by Friday morning Graham's INR will be moving rapidly towards the therapeutic target and at that time he can tell him to markedly reduce his dose.

Graham fails to keep his Friday morning appointment and upon contacting his office David is dismayed to be told that Graham has left the country for business and will not be returning until the evening of Sunday 12 March.

On Monday 13 March, Graham appears at the pharmacy at 9.00am, pleased with himself for having landed a lucrative business deal. He tells David not to worry. He just carried on taking the 10 mg each day at 6pm. Apart from some bleeding gums and a rather large bruise on his arm, where he must have banged it on something, he feels fine. When David takes Graham's INR, it has climbed to 8.0. Recognising that the patient is now at major risk of a bleed, David instructs Graham to stop the warfarin. David explains to Graham the risk he is now under, informs the GP and arranges for a venous sample to confirm the reading. Point-of-care testing may be inaccurate at this level and the patient's INR may be well in excess of this number. The *British National Formulary* (BNF) recommends stopping the warfarin and restarting when the INR falls below 5, provided there is no, or only minor, bleeding (Joint Formulary Committee, 2010).

Graham finally starts to appreciate the seriousness of the situation and agrees to keep all his future appointments as a priority. After 3 days, with daily INR checks, the level has dropped to 4.7. David gradually re-introduces the warfarin at a daily maintenance dose of 2 mg. David and Graham both recognise that they have had a narrow escape.

David's problems are not yet over. The laboratory results indicated an INR of 8.5. His Primary Care Organisation (PCO) require all critical incidents with warfarin to be reported to them directly and the local enhanced service (LES) which is part of his contract to provide this service for the PCO instructs that vitamin K as an antidote should be given orally to all patients with an INR of 8 or above without waiting for the results of the venous test.

1   To whom is David is responsible as a prescriber?
2   At what point in this patient's journey does David become responsible and therefore accountable for Graham's treatment? What considerations should David have taken into account before he prescribed for Graham?
3   What responsibility does David have to himself in this situation?
4   David has experienced a 'near miss' situation in his prescribing. What factors contributed to the error? How should David communicate this incident to the patient and other prescribers? What records does he need to keep? Is there anyone else that David needs to inform about what has happened? How can David reduce the risk of this kind of situation happening again?

Q1   To whom is David is responsible as a prescriber?

While David's overriding responsibility must be for the well-being of his patient, it is apparent from the above scenario that the actions taken by a prescriber have far wider implications. In the example above, David's actions have additionally impacted on the patient's GP, upon secondary care laboratory resources and have put him at odds with the advice of the haematologist. He has breached his terms of service with the PCO under the LES. If the patient had come to significant harm, the publicity could have discredited the programme to move the service out into the community. He could potentially have bought his profession into disrepute, as well as damaging his own reputation as prescriber and pharmacist. As an independent prescriber, David is professionally accountable for his prescribing decisions (Royal Pharmaceutical Society of Great Britain, 2007). He must make his own clinical assessment of the patient, establish his own diagnosis and formulate a plan for the clinical management of the patient. While he cannot delegate these responsibilities to another person, his employer has vicarious liability for his actions.

David breached one of the fundamental principles of prescribing, in that he prescribed outside his competency. He did not really understand the reason why Fennerty is only used in hospitalised patients where monitoring can be assured. His pharmacological knowledge of the medicine he was prescribing was woefully lacking. He failed to make a proper risk assessment of his initial decision to delay prescribing where the NICE indicates that prescribing an anticoagulant is appropriate. He was clearly acting outside his level of experience.

The Medicines Act 1968 was introduced by the Department of Health and Social Security following a review of legislation relating to medicines prompted by the thalidomide tragedy in the 1960s. It governs the manufacture and supply of medicines and divides them into three categories, Prescription Only Medicines (POM), Pharmacy Only Medicines (P) available for sale only through registered pharmacies and General Sales List (GSL) medicines, which can be purchased through non-pharmacy outlets. In 1999 the Supply and Administration of Medicines report (Department of Health, 1999) (the 'Crown report' – named after its author June Crown and not the Crown as in government) recommended that prescribing of POMs be extended under a supplementary role to professions other than doctors. These so called 'non-medical prescribers' initially included nurses and pharmacists. Section 63 of the Health and Social Care Act 2001 allowed the designation of new categories of prescriber, and set conditions for their prescribing. Amendments to the Prescription Only Medicines Order and changes to NHS regulations to allow the introduction of supplementary prescribing were laid before Parliament on 14 March 2003 and came into force on 4 April 2003. In May 2006, independent prescribing for both nurses and pharmacists was introduced. This expanded the ability to prescribe for any medical condition, but only within the individual's competency. In the above case study, David prescribed outside his competency and has therefore opened up the possibility of prosecution under criminal law. David is also vulnerable to prosecution under civil law by the patient for any consequences arising from his poor prescribing.

As a prescriber, David is subject to both criminal and civil law. Criminal law is the means by which the government identifies and criminalizes behaviour that is considered wrong, damaging to individuals or to society as a whole, or is otherwise unacceptable. It is enforced through the criminal justice system. This is the mechanism by which action is taken to deal with those suspected of committing offences and judgment is determined in the criminal courts. Civil law is enforced by private parties.

Prescribers need evidence that they maintain competency, in order to demonstrate that they have acted/continue to act as a professional, using the latest available evidence. Vicarious liability with the employer and personal insurance are essential for all prescribers. David's contract of employment and job description must cover the area in which he is working and should include prescribing as a named activity. The PCO will also have laid down service level agreements and specific competencies for each area of practice.

David has a responsibility for the security of prescriptions. He must record the first and last prescription 'pad number for each session, in case a prescription pad should go astray. Recording directly onto the surgery system ensures that a complete audit of his prescribing is maintained and can be accessed by the PCO for monitoring. David should follow best practice, by prescribing all four strengths of warfarin to avoid the need for alternate daily dosing (NPSA, 2007). He must be careful to write '5 milligrams' and '5 micrograms' in full to avoid dispensing errors, and ensure that the patient understands the difference between the two. In David's pharmacy, as an additional safeguard, the dispensing of any prescription written by David is carried out independently by an NVQ3 qualified dispenser and checked by a qualified accuracy checker to separate the functions of prescribing and dispensing.

Q2   At what point in this patient's journey does David become responsible, and therefore accountable, for Graham's treatment? What considerations should David have taken into account before he prescribed for Graham?

The decision to prescribe for a patient must be based on a combination of one's own competency in the clinical area, the ability to communicate and the consent of the patient. It is therefore apparent that the prescriber's responsibilities begin long before the patient walks through the door. Before commencing any service, it is essential that David can demonstrate his competency and defend his decisions.

At the point that David achieved his qualification, it is reasonable to expect that his knowledge was up to date or he would not have passed, but knowledge advances continuously and keeping current is a lifelong commitment. New medicines are licensed, existing medicines have their licences amended or withdrawn and protocols are updated. There is, of course, no shortage of ways to continue professional development, including short courses, literature searches and communication with colleagues and peers. It is essential each prescriber has a structure to their learning and that records of CPD are kept. The professional bodies have laid down the minimum standards each prescriber must meet and competency frameworks for non-medical prescribers are available (Department of Health, 2007).

To be competent, a prescriber must deliver a service that is effective, safe and of high quality. A competent practitioner will be able to defend all their decisions to their peers. Competency includes a combination of up-to-date knowledge, the ability to apply that knowledge, an understanding of patients and their motivations, and the ability to work inter-professionally, to provide a cost-effective service to achieve agreed national and local health outcomes. Competency frameworks are available from the National Prescribing Centre, which provides a structured approach to enable practitioners to audit their own performance against defined standards. To demonstrate his competency to prescribe in the area of anti-coagulation, David needs to ensure that he is familiar with national and local guidelines, and has a thorough knowledge of the pharmacology and disease processes for which he intends to prescribe (NPSA, 2007). Anticoagulants interact significantly with other medicines. The BNF provides a good summary of the key interactions. However, it may not provide sufficient detail on interactions with herbal and alternative medicines. David, specialising in the management of anticoagulation, will need to identify reliable, in-depth and up-to-date sources of information to support his practice.

The moment that David agrees to accept responsibility for treatment, a duty of care exists between himself and the patient. Fundamental to this is communication and, again, this begins before the first word is spoken. David needs to be appropriately dressed, ensure his surroundings are clean and tidy, and watch his body language. Luckily, in this scenario, David and Graham speak the same language, but this cannot be assumed and the interpretation of words needs careful consideration. Graham has already been told that warfarin 'thins his blood'. This may have created images of feeling cold, or not being able to do as much as he should be able to as his blood is not full strength. David would have the job of reassuring him that this is not the case, without undermining Graham's respect for his own GP, who may have used these words to convey the principle of anticoagulation in the limited time available. If Graham thinks that the pharmacist and GP are saying different things, he may be forced into believing one over the other. He may, of course, decide they are both wrong.

When David complied with the GP's request for anticoagulation, he needed to satisfy himself that anticoagulation was appropriate for this patient. NICE clinical guideline 36 lays out a stroke risk stratification to determine if the use of warfarin is appropriate (NICE, 2006). This is a useful tool, but David should have combined this with a complete patient history and a risk assessment of the patient sitting in front of him. Graham's hypertension, his poor compliance with his previous medication, his raised blood sugars and heroic alcohol intake, are all risk factors which may have contributed to his atrial fibrillation. Skilful negotiation would have been needed if the addition of a medicine with such a narrow therapeutic index as warfarin, was to be both safe and effective and improve his prognosis. David needed to ask himself what the chances were of Graham stopping drinking and smoking. Has he had or does he have any physical injury which would have increased the risk from anticoagulation? He mentioned paintballing with his mates for fun. David needed to address this and consider if Graham's work involved the risk of trauma. Being kicked by a horse is never a pleasant experience but whilst anticoagulated could prove fatal. David must recognise that the ramifications of treatment impact on more than just the individual sitting in front of him.

David also had the problem of Graham's current medication. Aspirin and warfarin are sometimes prescribed together under secondary care, but not under the NICE guidelines for atrial fibrillation (AF), as there is an increased risk of bleeding. Stopping the aspirin immediately, before the INR was therapeutic, would put the patient at increased risk. Calcium channel blockers increase the risk of AF and the rationale for the atenolol is uncertain. Clearly communication between David and the patient's GP would be essential at all times.

Q3   What responsibility does David have to himself in this situation?

David needs to ensure his personal protection when handling blood samples. This includes adequate hand-washing facilities and impervious wipeable worktops and floors. All staff handling blood need an up-to-date Hep B vaccination. Protective gloves must be worn at all times and changed between each patient. Professional, single-use lancets which prevent cross-contamination between patients are needed, together with safe disposal facilities to prevent needlestick injuries to David, his dispensary staff and cleaners. Test strips must be date checked and appropriately stored.

One aspect of prescribing which rarely gets consideration in the literature, but is of fundamental importance to the prescriber, is how prescribers can protect themselves emotionally. As a prescriber, you will see some patients on a regular basis, perhaps weekly or monthly for prolonged periods; others you will meet on a single occasion. When you speak to experienced prescribers they all have stories of self-doubt: 'Could I have done more for that patient? Should I have insisted that he was seen by a specialist or a generalist as a matter of urgency?' Your reaction to a particular situation may well be influenced by a previous communication with another professional, who may or may not have been as supportive as you feel they should have been or were even hostile to your intervention, as in David's case. Never get yourself into a position of regret. This may take great courage on your part, but if the worst case happens, can you look a widow or widower in the eye knowing that you could have done more? You could argue that this is just putting the patient at the centre of your work and this is true, but it actually goes one stage further than that, to acting in a way that you can live with yourself. Give your own well-being the same consideration as you give to your patients. This is an example of where it can be so helpful to have a mentor.

Q4   David has experienced a 'near miss' situation in his prescribing. What factors contributed to the error? How should David communicate this incident to the patient and other prescribers? What records does he need to keep? Is there anyone else that David needs to inform about what has happened? How can David reduce the risk of this kind of situation happening again?

In this case study David quickly realised that he had made a mistake in choosing an inappropriate loading regimen for this patient. He allowed pressure from the patient and the GP to influence his decision making. He found himself under a time pressure. He focused his attention on trying to placate the GP and by treating the disease and not the patient. He did not consider the pressures that either the GP or patient were under. David is not responsible for either the GP or the disease, but he is responsible for treating the patient safely and effectively. He is accountable to both the GP and the patient.

David needs to reflect on the undue influences he allowed the GP and the patient to have on his decision making and the factors in their relationships which led him into making a dubious decision. He needs to discuss these pressures with both the other parties who may not appreciate his position. He should reflect on his practice and record this in his CPD record. He failed to understand where his knowledge was insufficient for the actions he undertook (i.e. he acted outside his competence). He should document fully the events which led up to the error, and record in writing his communications with the doctor and patient.

David had the good sense to notify the GP of his error and to explain the situation to the patient. It appeared that Graham recognised ultimately that he too had some responsibility for his potentially fatal event. By implementing concordance, it doesn't mean that David gives into Graham and allows him to do anything he wants. David took some necessary steps, but failed to follow the locally agreed protocol for confirming high INR readings, even though he followed the BNF guidelines after correcting the situation. Local protocols may be based on the personal opinion of a local consultant and may vary from national evidence-based guidelines. This situation could contribute to inadvertent mistakes. The PCO should be made aware of this discrepancy, in David's case, and be able to defend their guidance. David has to be able to live with his decision and answer the question 'If I had followed local protocols, would the outcome have been different?' By accepting his error and taking steps to rectify the situation, he significantly reduced the potential for further action being taken against him. He did, however, also fail to inform his insurance company of the near miss and this could have led him into difficulty had the outcome not been so favourable. This could still happen in the future, should any long-term adverse consequences arise. His insurance company would have given him advice and guidance on admitting liability, which may affect their willingness to defend his case should litigation follow.

Had David attempted to cover up his mistakes and harm had come to the patient, David's position as an autonomous professional would have been indefensible.

While the exact nature of David's mistake may be unique, he is but one of many prescribers facing similar situations. The NPSA has a web-based facility that allows anonymous reporting to collate data on errors, near misses and fatal outcomes. Where common themes can be established, they publish evidence-based guidelines to reduce risk. In anticoagulation they have produced specific guidelines to make anticoagulation safer.

David would also benefit from having a mentor with whom he can meet regularly to discuss general issues related to prescribing. This should be someone David feels happy to talk to about any problems he is experiencing in his prescribing practice. This may be someone different from his clinical mentor who would be able to advise him on matters relating to anticoagulation. Some Trusts encourage new prescribers to 'buddy' up with another prescriber in this way. Some areas offer forums for prescribers.

Scenario conclusion

Several weeks later, David believes he and Graham have established a good rapport. The patients' review period has been extended to four weeks which he can accommodate into his lifestyle.

As Graham is leaving to collect his warfarin he turns to David:

> *By the way – good news they are going to try cardio version. They reckon I'll need weekly INR checks for at least seven weeks but they'll be lucky. If that doesn't work they are going to give me amiodarone – does that affect the warfarin? And next week I've booked the dentist for a tooth extraction, but that shouldn't affect anything as its not drugs is it? I could always try acupuncture if it hurts afterwards and I'm also thinking of starting cod liver oil for my joints. See you – I'm off for a pint.*

David believes (and hopes) that Graham is joking, but just in case he has been checking his facts. Cardioversion requires maintaining the patient at a higher INR target, amiodarone interacts with warfarin, as can cod liver oil, dental extraction may require dose adjustment. The biggest worry for David is that Graham may not behave any differently this time when frequent monitoring would again be required if any of those circumstances arose. What might David do differently should any (or all) of the above occur?

Prescribing pitfalls

- Don't allow yourself to be pressurised by patients, colleagues, receptionists, relatives or anyone else to prescribe outside areas in which you feel competent or that take you outside your legal boundaries.
- Don't make assumptions about your insurance cover – check the details in relation to prescribing.
- Avoid taking on the patient's burden – if you are feeling weighed down seek help.
- Never attempt to cover up mistakes. Be honest with all affected parties.
- When taking blood samples from patients it is necessary to inform your insurance company.
- Never open the door to a patient while wearing a pair of rubber gloves. Always put on a clean pair after they are with you.

Top tips

- Keep up to date with guidelines. Make the most of websites such as NICE, NELM and NPC, who filter information and send you validated links.
- Record everything you do, whether it is issuing a prescription, giving advice or referring.
- Follow your gut instinct when dealing with patients. You get a lot from body language and signals that your conscious may not register.
- Prepare well in advance – the patient contact is the last step.
- Protect yourself – your mental health as well as your patient's health is important. Find a 'buddy' with whom you can talk through issues.
- Accept you will not always be right. Reflect on your practice. The person who never made a mistake never made anything.
- Use competency frameworks if relevant to your role and follow your professional body code of ethics. Read them more than once.
- Be prepared to justify, using the evidence base where possible, all prescribing decisions. Ensure you act in a way that a competent prescriber using due care would do or follow well-recognised school of thought so that your actions would be supported by your colleagues. Read the Bolam case.
- Think outside the box. Who else will your actions affect? What other actions do you need to take? What could the patient be doing to enhance/disrupt treatment?
- Anticoagulants are few in number, but interact with a wide range of prescribed and over the counter medicines and complementary and

alternative therapies. A thorough patient history and current medicine regimen needs to be established before agreeing to treat these patients. It is important to establish a rapport and trust with the patient so that they will consult you before self-medicating, come and see you as soon as any medication is changed or doses adjusted, and be honest with you about missed doses and alcohol intake. Patients under the care of renal, hepatic or haemophilia centres may have very different monitoring and dosing requirements.

References

Baglin T, Keeling D, Watson H (2005). Guidelines on oral anticoagulation (warfarin): third edition – 2005 update. *British Society for Haematology* 132: 277–285.

Department of Health (1999) Review of prescribing, supply and administration of medicines. Available at: www.dh.gov.uk/en/Publicationsandstatistics/Publications/PublicationsPolicyAndGuidance/DH_4077151 [Accessed 20 December 2009].

Department of Health (2007) Continuing professional development. Available at: www.dh.gov.uk/prod_consum_dh/groups/dh_digitalassets/@dh/@en/documents/digitalasset/dh_4074371.pdf [Accessed 20 December 2009].

Department of Health (2008) Delivering care closer to home: meeting the challenge. Available at: www.dh.gov.uk/prod_consum_dh/groups/dh_digitalassets/@dh/@en/documents/digitalasset/dh_086051.pdf [Accessed 20 December 2009].

Joint Formulary Committee (2010) *BNF: British National Formulary 60*. London: British Medical Association and Royal Pharmaceutical Society of Great Britain, October.

NICE (National Institute for Health and Clinical Excellence) (2006) Clinical Guideline 36, Atrial Fibrillation: The management of atrial fibrillation. Available at: www.nice.org.uk/nicemedia/pdf/CG036niceguideline.pdf [Accessed 20 December 2009].

NPSA (National Patient Safety Agency) (2007) Actions that can make anticoagulant therapy safer: Work competences. Available at: www.nrls.npsa.nhs.uk/resources/?entryid45=61790&q=0%c2%acanticoagulant%c2%ac [Accessed 20 December 2009].

Royal Pharmaceutical Society of Great Britain (2007) Professional Standards and Guidance for Pharmacist Prescribers. Available at: www.rpsgb.org/pdfs/coepsgpharmpresc.pdf [Accessed 20 December 2009].

Further reading/websites of interest

Barnes J, Anderson L, Phillipson J (2003). Herbal interactions. *Pharmaceutical Journal* 270: 118–121.

Bolam vs Friern Management Committee (1957) http://oxcheps.new.ox.ac.uk/casebook/Resources/BOLAMV_1%20DOC.pdf [Accessed 20 December 2009].

Health and Social Care Act 2001. www.opsi.gov.uk/Acts/acts2001/en/ukpgaen_20010015_en_1 [Accessed 20 December 2009].

Medicines Act 1968. www.opsi.gov.uk/RevisedStatutes/Acts/ukpga/1968/cukpga_19680067_en_1 [Accessed 20 December 2009].

National Prescribing Centre (2006) Maintaining competency in prescribing. www.keele.ac.uk/schools/pharm/npcplus/prescribing/documents/pharmacist_comp_framework_Oct06.pdf [Accessed 20 December 2009].

Royal Pharmaceutical Society of Great Britain (2007) Professional standards and guidance for pharmacist prescribers. www.rpsgb.org/pdfs/coepsgpharmpresc.pdf [Accessed 20 December 2009].

Mind map

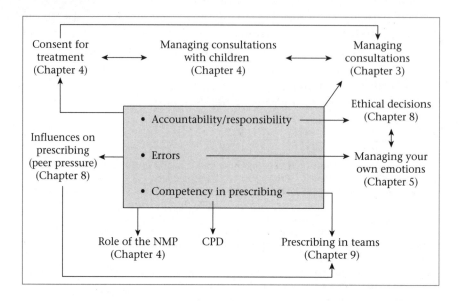

Consent for treatment (Chapter 4) ←→ Managing consultations with children (Chapter 4) ←→ Managing consultations (Chapter 3)

- Accountability/responsibility → Ethical decisions (Chapter 8)

Influences on prescribing (peer pressure) (Chapter 8) ← • Errors → Managing your own emotions (Chapter 5)

- Competency in prescribing

Role of the NMP (Chapter 4)   CPD   Prescribing in teams (Chapter 9)

3

Taking a good history

Jane Colbert

Learning outcomes

After completing this chapter you will be able to:

- identify what constitutes the 'essential elements' of good history taking;
- list the fundamental points to cover when taking an accurate medication history;
- describe strategies for prioritising in a consultation.

Introduction

This chapter is about exploring a given consultation with the patient, and as such is not designed to teach consultation skills. There are many excellent books on the subject, some of which are listed in the further reading section. The chapter uses a scenario to identify some of the key points to think about when carrying out a consultation during which you may consider prescribing. The chapter focuses on the sometimes tricky issue of prioritising prescribing decisions based on the information available. It also questions how far history taking should go and to what extent the patient's agenda should be considered.

The scenario presented is probably one of the most common encountered in actual practice: the 'busy' patient with an agenda that does not readily lend itself to a 'brief consultation' before prescribing. It is only the unwise or foolhardy prescriber that would consider putting pen to pad (or issuing a computer-generated prescription) before making sure a thorough history is taken. As the scenario demonstrates, the potential for problems is vast. Here we shall address the problems inherent with trying to prescribe 'piecemeal'.

Prescriber

Julie Radley has been qualified as a nurse for 15 years. After a brief spell working in hospital, she moved into primary care where she has worked as a 'practice nurse' for the same single-handed general practitioner (GP) for 13 years. Last year her 'regular' GP retired and the patient list was taken over by the Primary Care Trust (PCT) with all services relocated to a new Healthy Living Centre two miles down the road. As a consequence, Julie became part of a team of four nurses, all of whom are prescribers. She completed her prescribing qualification earlier this year and, to her surprise, did quite well on the course and has enjoyed a cautious start to her prescribing career. The other nurses in the practice have specialised in long-term conditions, but Julie prefers to see minor ailments and family planning-related problems. In her previous role, she did deal with asthma and diabetic patients extensively, but now chooses to leave this to the other nurses.

Patient background

Sally Harris is a 44-year-old woman who is an infrequent visitor to the surgery. She works as a dentist in the next town and is a 'no nonsense' kind of person. Life has not been too kind to Sally of late. Her husband of almost 25 years left her 18 months ago after admitting to a long-term affair with a work colleague. Shortly after this, her mother died unexpectedly, leaving her father alone. Sally, an only child, is his sole support. Her father currently lives 35 miles away and Sally, in an attempt to minimise the travelling, has been hoping to persuade him to move closer to her.

Sally has two daughters, both of whom are away at university, studying medicine. She does not get to see them much, although she supports them financially as her ex husband now has a new family.

On the surface Sally has coped well with all these changes to her life. She lives alone in a house which still has a sizeable mortgage. She has started to see an old male friend from her past, but insists it is 'just for company'.

Name: Sally Harris
DOB: 3/6/*forty-four years ago*
Occupation: Dentist

Past medical history

Appendectomy at age 10
Termination of pregnancy at age 17
Back pain at age 22
SVD live infant (female) at age 23
Anterior uveitis (iritis) at age 26
SVD live infant (female) at age 25
Chest infection at age 28
Asthma at age 30
Iritis at age 35
Back pain at age 35
Iritis at age 40
Problems with sleeping/anxiety at age 42
Anxiety at age 43

Current medication

Microgynon 30 (levonorgestrel 150 micrograms, ethinylestradiol
    30 micrograms) – *last dispensed 1 year ago*
Salbutamol inhaler 100 micrograms – *last dispensed 9 months ago*

Past medication

Pred Forte eye drops (prednisolone acetate 1%) – *last prescribed
    9 months ago*
Cyclopentolate eye drops (single use) 1% – *last prescribed 9 months
    ago*
Betnesol eye ointment (betamethasone sodium phosphate 0.1%)
    – *last prescribed 9 months ago*
Meloxicam 15 mg one daily – *last prescribed 2 years ago*
Lansoprazole 15 mg one daily – *last prescribed 2 years ago*

continued overleaf

Disease monitoring

PEFR: 460 mL/min assessed *2 years ago*
BMI: 29 *calculated today*
Blood pressure: *Today* 136/82 mmHg; *1 year ago* 136/82 mmHg;
    2 years ago 134/82 mmHg

Social history

Separated from husband *18 months ago*
Occasional smoker (recorded 3 years ago). Today – non-smoker
Alcohol 18 units a week
No exercise

Scenario

Sally arrives in the consultating room, clearly irritated, announcing *'I'm going on holiday tomorrow and I haven't even packed yet.'* It appears that Sally has only come to see Julie because an appointment wasn't available with her usual doctor. She is clearly upset because she has had to wait for a long time in the waiting room. Julie apologises (feeling slightly guilty at the extra time she took with Mrs Bennett earlier that morning which did make her subsequent appointments run later than usual). Sally perches uneasily on the edge of the chair. She rarely comes to the surgery and has been irritated to find that the one time she does require an appointment, she is unable see her preferred GP (there is a two-week wait for a 'routine' appointment it appears) and that she has wasted precious time sitting in the waiting room. 'If I ran my dental practice like this . . . I would be out of business' she finishes.

A brief scan of Sally's records shows Julie that Sally's general health appears good for her age. As she rarely attends the surgery, there is little information available on both written notes and the computer screen. She has had letters recently calling her for asthma check and cervical smear, both of which are still outstanding.

Julie starts the consultation by asking Sally how she can help her today. The reply is

I need my Pill for the next year and I also want a repeat of my eye drops and salbutamol – just in case – as I am off on holiday tomorrow. Last

time I was on holiday I had a flare up of my iritis and I had an awful problem getting effective treatment. In the end I had to come home early.

Julie has a tried and tested method for progressing her consultations. As this is the first time she has met Sally, Julie does a quick review of Sally's asthma and contraceptive history to which Sally gives clipped, one-word answers. However, in this 'review' Julie establishes that Sally had her last attack of iritis 4 years ago and that although her back has been painful, it is effectively managed with 'painkillers'. Julie leaves it at that in an attempt to make up time. She then begins her medication history taking by reviewing Sally's Microgynon use and establishes that she had started her last pack of pills two weeks ago. She also establishes that salbutamol use is minimal, last being used after exposure to cat fur two months ago. Prior to that, it was used 'only rarely'. Julie feels that she is making progress. She finishes off her consultation by enquiring about Sally's allergies and smoking status. Sally still has no known allergies, but confesses that she has started smoking in the evenings again after having given up for 3 years. Julie senses that Sally is embarrassed by confessing this and decides not to push this on this occasion and threaten their newly developing rapport. This is something she can tackle the next time she sees this patient.

Having completed her history taking and gathered her information Julie now contemplates prescribing for Sally.

Reflective questions

1   What is Sally's agenda for this consultation? How does this differ from Julie's and what challenges does this present Julie as a relatively inexperienced prescriber?
2   How might Sally's 'medical' background influence Julie's decision making?
3   What points in Sally's medical history is it important for Julie to explore in *this* consultation?
4   What information does Julie need to explore when taking a medication history from Sally in *this* consultation?
5   How can Julie prioritise her approach to this consultation? What does she need to do today to help Sally? What should Julie include when considering her 'safety net'?

Q1   What is Sally's agenda for this consultation? How does this differ from Julie's and what challenges does this present Julie as a relatively inexperienced prescriber?

Sally has come to the surgery today with a stated agenda: to leave the surgery with a prescription for both her contraceptive pill and also the 'standby' medicines needed for this holiday. The last-minute rushed nature of her consultation and her irritation at not getting what she wanted at a time of her choosing, may be quite genuine and Julie really has no choice but to take this at face value.

Patients may use a number of 'mechanisms' to obtain medication and these may not always be as straightforward as they first appear. Sally may be using the extra pressure inherent in a pre-holiday consultation to avoid the asthma checkup and smear test which she has been called for. This could be because she views them as a waste of time, or simply because she has fears about their results: it is impossible to say. Sally may have remortgaged her house and made declarations on her form which would explain her reticence to attend the surgery or have any official diagnoses made that may limit her ability to continue working or affect her pension provision, for example.

A consultation can be a patient's way of engaging with health professionals about matters that they consider more difficult to discuss. Sally's records show that she has experienced anxiety and sleep problems in the past. There was no prescription given for these but Julie could have enquired about them in her history taking. Of course, Sally may deny a problem, but at least Julie could have documented that she had asked. There is also the issue that Sally has taken up smoking again after 3 years. This begs the question why?

Julie's agenda must include taking a history that is comprehensive enough to safely and effectively manage this patient. This management may include writing a prescription. There are different models for history taking and it is important that each prescriber has his or her own structure/ method for approaching this. Although it won't be necessary to cover every part of the structure on every occasion, it is vitally important to focus on the key parts that enable safe and effective patient management to inform decisions made. Julie could argue that in Sally's case 'nothing has changed since last time' and that issuing repeat prescriptions for all her regular medication is appropriate.

Julie appears to have carried out 'selected highlights' from her consultation 'menu'. However, this may have been driven more by her own comfort zone than her desire to take an adequate history. Like many prescribers, Julie may be unfamiliar with some of the medicines that her patient is taking and yet she is being asked to take full responsibility for the prescribing of these. As a non-medical prescriber, she will have been taught that she must only prescribe within her area of competence. Julie might reasonably view herself as competent to prescribe asthma medication and the contraceptive pill for Sally, but is she really competent to prescribe the eye preparations? If Julie decides to write a prescription for the eye medication and something goes wrong, she alone would be fully responsible in law for that prescribing. One could therefore argue that Julie should have asked more questions about this aspect of Sally's history and the medication used to control it. Perhaps Julie hoped to delegate this aspect of Sally's prescribing to another colleague. Is this fair? Perhaps it is, if the colleague has more experience. Asking a GP colleague to sign a prescription for the eye preparations, when Julie herself has seen the patient, could be seen as negligent and may not relieve Julie of her responsibilities in law.

Q2   How might Sally's 'medical' background influence Julie's decision making?

Sally's professional background might put Julie under extra pressure to prescribe, or at the very least to admit that she is uncertain about something. Alternatively, Julie might be lulled into a false sense of security by Sally's medical background. Sally will be a prescriber herself, so surely she would understand her own medication? Sally should know not to put another healthcare professional under pressure to prescribe and yet she is doing this unconsciously (or otherwise). Healthcare professionals should not be assumed to have any particular specialist knowledge or understanding, nor any magical powers that make them more compliant with medication than any other patient. It is Julie who is taking responsibility for what she prescribes, not Sally.

Q3   What points in Sally's medical history is it important for Julie to explore in *this* consultation?

From the briefest of history given here, it is clear that there are many issues that need to be addressed before any decision on treatment or a prescription may be considered. As Julie is not familiar with some of the medications Sally has been given in the past, she may not fully understand the reasons for Sally's request. A brief perusal of the *British National Formulary* (BNF) or computer search will help to explain the medications and the indications for prescribing these items (Joint Formulary Committee, 2010). Ideally, this should be undertaken before a patient arrives, as it is important for prescribers not to ignore the 'unknown' medicines or underlying medical conditions that patients have. As a minimum, is it important to consider 'what effect will what I prescribe have on these medicines/conditions?' and likewise 'what effect do these medicines/conditions have on my prescribing?'

Julie has three main aspects to consider today: the request for the contraceptive, the asthma medication and the eye preparations. She has to determine whether anything has changed in Sally's history since each of these items was last prescribed that may affect the safe and effective use of these items by this patient.

Sally has made an appointment for a repeat prescription for her contraceptive pill. Her records state that she was last issued a prescription one year ago. A full sexual health history could be warranted, although this may need to be approached with tact. At an absolute minimum, the continued need for contraception should be established today, together with Sally's compliance with her current regimen. Julie does not appear to have enquired about over the counter (OTC), herbal or complementary medications that Sally might be taking. Sally might have started St John's wort, for example, and this could have implications for the efficacy of her contraceptive cover. Given Sally's age (and recent smoking status) a change to another method of contraception may be preferable for the future. Julie may choose to mention this today and issue only a short supply of contraceptive 'cover', using the issue of the overdue smear as a device by which she will ensure Sally's return, when the focus can be solely on her sexual health.

Sally has requested a prescription for ocular medication prior to holiday. This is not an unusual or unreasonable request, but may pose a problem for a prescriber, especially if the medications in question have previously been prescribed by a specialist (an ophthalmologist in this case). This poses an additional problem for Julie (as it would for many prescribers) as medications of this type are usually outside the average prescriber's remit and must never be prescribed as routine. Iritis is a condition that can flare without warning and there is certainly an argument in favour of a prescription being issued in order for treatment to be instigated promptly before requesting the patient attend the local ophthalmic department to confirm the diagnosis. It is also worth remembering that medications of this type may quickly go out of date in between 'flares'. Patients, having been at the mercy of the local ophthalmic hospital casualty department, may well be reluctant to travel abroad (Julie needs to establish if Sally is travelling abroad) without their supplies. Julie needs to combine a good review of the specialist's communication with the practice together with careful questioning of Sally and, if possible, advice from more experienced colleagues (without necessarily unfairly passing the buck). Julie has also to weigh up the consequences of not prescribing.

Sally has also requested a salbutamol inhaler, yet has not attended the asthma clinic. A brief glance at the screen would suggest minimal usage. At the same time, as the prescriber, Julie may feel a duty of care to check her asthma before issuing a prescription. Here, the short-term 'fix' of prescribing an inhaler may prevent Sally attending the asthma clinic for many months to come. Yet again the consequences of not prescribing must be considered.

There are many areas within this scenario that are ripe for exploration (sleeping, anxiety, smoking) but if Sally has no intention of having these areas explored, there is little the prescriber can do. There is no right or wrong solution to this problem and each prescriber would tackle this slightly differently. What is not a wise option, however, is to view this particular scenario as 'a nice quick appointment' – a pill check and a repeat prescription. To do this would be to ignore potential pitfalls in the consultation that may eventually lead to a negligence claim. This is not wishing to be alarmist, but from a practical viewpoint, prescribers need to be constantly aware of the bigger picture. Can Julie honestly say from the information she has acquired in the scenario to date, that Sally is not pregnant, for example?

Q4   What information does Julie need to explore when taking a medication history from Sally in *this* consultation?

Julie needs to establish whether the medication that she has listed for Sally is the medication that she is actually taking. She needs to ask about each medication in turn and ask Sally what problem she takes the medication for (unless she has expressed this knowledge already). This also involves questioning about exactly how she takes each medicine and whether, in her opinion, the medication is working. She should also enquire about any changes that might have occurred since taking the medication. Julie is actually looking for evidence of 'side-effects', but using these words in particular can sometimes limit how people answer. Patients often understand a side-effect to mean something 'undesirable' or 'unacceptable'. As a consequence, for example, patients may not report drowsiness that persists into the next day as an unacceptable side-effect if they had previously encountered difficulties with sleeping. The common problem of 'cough' associated with ACE inhibitors is frequently underreported and as such is often not perceived to be a 'side-effect' by the patient.

Asking patients what they take their medication for and whether it is working gives the prescriber information about the patient's understanding of the medication and the management of their condition. Julie needs to find out if Sally takes medication from any other source. Perhaps she has prescribed medication for herself (the dental surgery is a potential source of medication for patients generally, although it has a slightly different connotation in this scenario!).

We have already mentioned that Julie should have asked about OTC and alternative medication. Many people do not view the 'Pill' as 'medication' and, as a prescriber, you may have to be mindful of this in your questioning. Medication bought OTC, via the internet or brought home from abroad is becoming increasingly common, and should form a natural part of the medication history sequence.

All of this information is useful when considering management options and/or the addition of other medication. If Sally uses medication OTC which might be constipating, Julie needs to be aware of this in case she also wishes to prescribe something that has this effect. The fact that patients choose to take OTC medication may be in response to poorly controlled symptoms, or to try to cope with side-effects of 'prescribed' medication. Each part of the medication history adds a vital piece of the puzzle.

Q5   How can Julie prioritise her approach to this consultation? What does she need to do today to help Sally? What should Julie include when considering her 'safety net'?

Today, Julie must establish Sally's need for contraception and, if required, a 'suitable' prescription given for a duration of time required to ensure continuous cover. For the future, she will need to encourage Sally to attend for a smear test, but most importantly, discuss at length her ongoing contraceptive requirements, with a view to prescribing an alternative method of contraception. Dependent on Sally's answers, this may need to be included in the consultation today.

Julie needs to make a decision as to how to manage the request for the ocular preparations. The good prescriber would find out as much as possible about the condition and preparations, apply this to Sally's situation and seek advice from colleagues. At the end of the day, the prescriber must act in the patient's best interests. If to prescribe would be dangerous for the patient, because it is outside Julie's competency, she must decline, but she does have a professional responsibility to find someone who will be able to help Sally.

The asthma situation is perhaps more tricky. Julie may have the competency – but does she have the time in this 'mixed agenda' consultation? A full asthma assessment is clearly impractical, but somehow, Sally does need to be encouraged to come back. Perhaps a double appointment at the time of the next Pill check may be the way forward? Then she could combine two problems within one consultation. Sally's response to this proposal will really inform how Julie goes forward.

Scenario conclusion

Julie did manage to persuade Sally to return after her holiday and booked her for a double appointment. After all the fuss, Sally had actually forgotten to take her Pill with her on holiday and this had led to a 'bit of a scare'. By the time she met with Julie again, she was extremely motivated to use a different method of contraception. Sally decided that given the nature of her busy life, the coil would be her preferred method for the next few years.

Julie has recently undertaken some more training which has enabled her to reflect on her consultation skills again. She is happy with her basic consultation structure and style but she is becoming more skilled at including the patient in the decision-making process and has been looking at decision-making tools to help her and her patients with this aspect of the consultation.

Following a clinical meeting in which this scenario was discussed, the surgery as a whole recognised that they have little or no expertise in eye problems. As a result, the local ophthalmologist has been invited to attend one of the clinical meetings, to give the staff an update on ocular conditions and common medications. One of the GPs has offered to write a protocol for managing eye conditions within the general practice setting in conjunction with the hospital consultant. For her part, Julie has attended the ophthalmology clinic, sitting in on a session with the nurse consultant. She now has an expert practitioner within her 'network' whom she can contact in the future for advice.

Sally did reluctantly agree to an asthma check-up. Her asthma is well controlled with only very occasional salbutamol use. It appears that Sally had heard that the surgery was only carrying out asthma checks to achieve Quality and Outcome Framework (QOF) points which was one excuse for her reticence to attend. Julie was able to explain the rationale behind the Framework and while Sally isn't entirely convinced to date, she does appreciate that it is ultimately her choice whether to attend or not in the future.

In conclusion, each consultation may be viewed as a puzzle, which ultimately will lead to a decision being made – either to prescribe or to give advice, or both. Given that 'prescribing' represents the end part of this process, which also has an outcome associated with the greatest potential for an adverse event, we must consider very carefully the strategies we choose to employ in order to reach a safe and effective decision.

Prescribing pitfalls

- Don't ignore the 'unknown medicine'. You need to find out more about the 'canvas' on which you will be prescribing before you start. Ideally you should do this before the patient arrives.
- Don't follow your 'history template' doggedly at the expense of more focused questions.
- Avoid haphazard history taking or not covering each subject in sufficient depth. In some situations, you may just have to deal with the most urgent problem on that day only and plan for the next time. Remember to record your decisions and plans in the patient notes.
- Never make assumptions about pregnancy – ask each time. Consider the consequences of prescribing for a newly pregnant woman when you didn't ask the question.
- Do not be tempted to prescribe outside your area of competence. It can be a tough call, but at the end of the day, which is the best course of action for the patient? If you aren't competent, then you are not safe; however, you must always consider the consequences of not prescribing.

Top tips

- Accept that your first tentative steps on your prescribing journey will be just that – 'tentative'. Don't be too hard on yourself, and instead view any anxiety that it provokes as positive. You are really thinking about each and every decision now.
- Never be afraid to admit to patients that you need to check something you are unsure of or if you do not understand their problem fully. Most patients will view this as you being thorough. Don't worry that patients will view this negatively as a lack of knowledge. You are being a true professional by exercising a duty of care to your patients. That is all that counts.

- It is possible to identify gaps in your knowledge and put steps in place to reduce the possibility of errors. Do this before you start prescribing and review this constantly throughout your prescribing career.
- Never underestimate the importance of taking a good history, even if you are an expert in your field. Make a personalised template to guide your history taking to ensure that you are being as thorough as you can possibly be.
- Fully document your findings, examinations and recommendations. If you didn't record it, you didn't do it, see it, ask it or even consider it.
- Be aware that what you consider as medication may not be what your patient considers as 'medication'.
- Always be aware of the 'hidden' problems that can catch you out – allergies, OTC medicines or internet medicines, underlying 'active' disease, co-morbidities, pregnancy, among others.
- Each consultation will have two perfectly valid agendas – yours and that of your patient. Try to find the middle ground and negotiate how best to proceed.
- Patients are complicated. Each has his or her own individual story to tell and rarely do they present with just one problem. If you are not prepared to dig deeper, you will only see the surface of the problem and miss out the issues that lie beneath.
- Ask yourself this question after each consultation: 'Have I taken a good enough history and do I have all the facts to enable me to prescribe safely and effectively for this patient?' If you are unable to answer this question satisfactorily, you are on shaky ground. Go back to square one.

Reference

Joint Formulary Committee (2010) *BNF: British National Formulary 60*. London: British Medical Association and Royal Pharmaceutical Society of Great Britain.

Further reading/websites of interest

Bickley L (2009) *Bates' Guide to Physical Examination and History Taking*, 10th edn. Philadelphia: Lippincott, Williams and Wilkins.
Calgary–Cambridge (2010) Calgary-Cambridge Guide to the medical interview: communication process. Available at: www.gp-training.net/training/communication_skills/calgary/guide.htm [Accessed June 2010].
Cox N and Roper T (2005) *Clinical Skills*. Oxford: Oxford University Press.
Douglas D, Nicol F and Robertson C (2009) *Macleod's Clinical Examination*, 12th edn. Edinburgh: Churchill Livingstone Elsevier.
Gleadle J (2007) *History and Examination at a Glance*, 2nd edn. Oxford: Wiley-Blackwell.

Robinson A, Thomson R (2001). Variability in patient preferences for participating in medical decision making: implication for the use of decision support tools. *Quality in Health Care* 10(Suppl): i34–i38.

Shwartz M (2010) *Textbook of Physical Diagnosis: History and examination*, 6th edn. Philadelphia: Saunders.

Silverman JD, Kurtz SM and Draper J (2005) *Skills for Communicating with Patients*, 2nd edn. Oxford: Radcliffe Medical Press.

Mind map

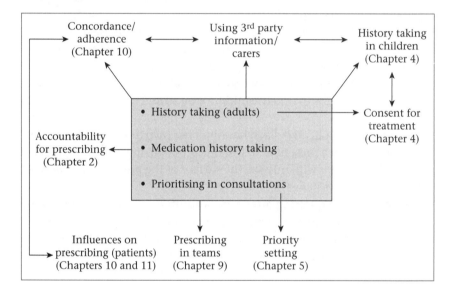

4

Consultations involving children

Angela Black

Learning outcomes

After completing this chapter you will be able to:

- identify the key points required when taking a history for a child with complex needs;
- outline the key factors underlying the process of gaining consent when prescribing for children;
- confirm the principles of deciding who has parental responsibility.

Introduction

Chapter 3 dealt with some of the challenges inherent in a consultation with an adult. This chapter looks at how good history taking can be achieved when the patient is a child. Gaining accurate information from a third party and putting that information into context is important in many situations, not just when dealing with children, and requires particular skill. This scenario also considers the difficulties that arise if, as in this case, the patient's parents have different wishes in relation to the child's treatment. This also raises the issue of gaining consent.

Prescriber

Ailsa Hughes is a physiotherapist who specialises in working with children with neurological conditions. She recently qualified as a non-medical prescriber to enable her, as part of a team, to work towards decreasing spasticity and pain in children with neurological conditions such as cerebral palsy. Medicine management is one method of treatment available to practitioners involved with children with cerebral palsy and is used in conjunction with other therapy modalities. In a report published in 2007 Rosenbaum *et al.* stated that:

> Cerebral palsy describes a group of permanent disorders of the development of movement and posture, causing activity limitations that are attributed to non-progressive disturbances that occurred in the developing foetal or infant brain. The motor disorders of cerebral palsy are often accompanied by disturbances of sensation, perception, cognition, communication, and behaviour, by epilepsy, and by secondary musculoskeletal problems.

Patient background

Lucie Bothy was born at 28 weeks gestation by caesarean section as her mother had pre-eclampsia (high blood pressure of pregnancy). Immediately after birth, Lucie was very unwell and needed to be ventilated on the special care baby unit (SCBU) for six weeks. In the early period she had several seizures, which were managed with medication. An early brain scan showed some areas of damage, but her prognosis was unknown. She was fed initially via a nasogastric tube, but once off the ventilator learnt to take a bottle and gradually put on weight. She was discharged home aged 38 weeks, still requiring oxygen.

As she was often unsettled and jumpy she remained on anti-epileptic medication. Lucie was prescribed phenytoin (one agent used where there is a risk of seizure recurrence in neonates).

Because of her stormy neonatal period and uncertain prognosis, Lucie was referred to the children's therapy team aged three months and was seen regularly by the appropriate members of the team, including the physiotherapist. Lucie was always a sickly baby; however, this worsened at six months of age. Following investigations, she was diagnosed with gastro-oesophageal reflux disorder (GORD) and was started on ranitidine (this H_2-receptor antagonist is widely used to heal gastric and duodenal ulcers, but can also be used to relieve dyspepsia and GORD). Overall, her general development was slow and she required support to help with her movement development. Initially, Lucie found it hard to hold her head up in different positions. Under the guidance of the therapy team, her parents worked with her every day, encouraging her movement skills, which gradually began to develop.

As Lucie began to move more, it became obvious that her muscle tone was increasing. Spasticity is where the muscle tone increases (there is a velocity-dependent increase in resistance to passive movement), which in turn makes movement and handling more difficult as the child becomes stiffer. For Lucie, spasticity was impacting on all aspects of her functioning, so at 18 months she was referred to Ailsa for an assessment.

Summary sheet with background information

Name: Lucie Bothy
Age: *18 months*

Past medical history

Born at 28 weeks gestation
Ventilated for six weeks on SCBU
Discharged home at 38 weeks requiring oxygen
Gastro-oesophageal reflux disorder (GORD) diagnosed age six
    months

Current medication

Phenytoin suspension 30 mg/5 mL. Dose: 60 mg twice daily
    (5 mg/kg twice daily)
Ranitidine oral solution 75 mg/5 mL. Dose: 24 mg (1.6 mL) twice
    daily (2 mg/kg twice a day)

Monitoring

Current weight: 12 kg
Current height: 80 cm

Social history

Lucie is an only child
She lives with mother and spends alternate weekends with her
    father
Her parents have recently divorced

Scenario

Ailsa has been asked to meet Lucie and her parents to discuss the possibility of prescribing baclofen to reduce spasticity. This drug is most commonly prescribed for spasm in children as it is associated with lower levels of addiction than diazepam, a possible alternative. Baclofen is licensed for children over one year and is available as a solution.

Ailsa is aware that Lucie's parents have just undergone a fairly acrimonious divorce and that Lucie now divides her time between two homes.

Both parents arrive together for today's appointment. In the consultation they report that Lucie has not had a seizure for three months and she is otherwise well. They describe what life with Lucie is like for each of them at the moment. Lucie remains totally dependent on her parents for all aspects of her daily life. Her mother looks after Lucie most of the time and is finding it increasingly difficult to carry out everyday activities such as nappy changing. She also describes how Lucie tends to stiffen when she is being put into her chair/car seat and that she is finding it more of a challenge to be able to position Lucie well. Her father, who looks after Lucie for shorter periods at the weekend, is not finding it difficult to position Lucie. However, her mother feels that this is because he has less equipment at his house (as he sees Lucie for shorter periods) and that he is physically stronger than she is. Her father feels that her mother is not being strict enough and that Lucie is 'playing her up'.

Reflective questions

1   What expectations might Lucie's parents have of Ailsa in this situation?
2   What information should Ailsa gather as part of her consultation with Lucie's parents? How much information will come from the parental assessment of the situation and how much will be contributed indirectly from Lucie herself? At what age would you consider asking the views of the child directly? How should Ailsa approach gaining consent for treatment?
3   How can Ailsa ensure that the parents understand the possible benefits or risks involved in starting to use baclofen for Lucie?
4   How could Ailsa involve Lucie's parents in monitoring her response to treatment?

Q1   What expectations might Lucie's parents have of Ailsa in this situation?

The parents may question if Ailsa is the most appropriate person to be prescribing for Lucie. Ailsa will need to explain to the parents her role in the team and what skills she has as a supplementary non-medical prescriber. Traditionally it is the doctor's role to prescribe medication, but in this case, the physiotherapist is in an ideal position as a supplementary prescriber to be able to closely monitor and assess the effects of the medication on the child and adjust the dosage appropriately. To enable Ailsa to prescribe for Lucie, she will need to write and agree a clinical management plan (CMP) with the child's paediatrician (who is acting as independent prescriber in this tripartite arrangement) and gain the parents' verbal agreement. (These discussions and the parental agreement should be recorded in the patient notes.) The use of a CMP fulfils the legal obligations for supplementary prescribing and ensures that good communication is developed between all those involved in the child's care.

The CMP is not the same as a care plan, but can form part of it. The CMP will specify the medicines that Ailsa can prescribe for Lucie for which conditions and will also state the dose range and when referral back to the independent prescriber (in this case the paediatrician) is appropriate. It will detail any local or national guidance which is applied in this case. Review dates are also included. More details about CMPs can be found in the further reading.

A general issue that Ailsa needs to address with Lucie's parents early on in her relationship with them is the use of medicines 'off label' for children. If she was also prescribing unlicensed medicines she would need to cover this too. This is discussed in more detail in the continuation of this scenario in Chapter 6.

Q2   What information should Ailsa gather as part of her consultation with Lucie's parents? How much information will come from the parental assessment of the situation and how much will be contributed indirectly from Lucie herself? At what age would you consider asking the views of the child directly? How should Ailsa approach gaining consent for treatment?

Ailsa will need to gather information from both parents. She will need to ask both parents about their main concerns regarding Lucie. These will initially inform Ailsa about their expectations of both her as the prescriber and the proposed treatment. In this case, both parents may express different views to which Ailsa will need to respond. Lucie has complex needs and is unable to express herself verbally; however, she is able to respond to pain/discomfort by crying and to express her happiness and general well-being by smiling. Her parents, being close to her, are the best people to interpret these subtle responses. Her parents will also know what is 'normal' behaviour and movement for Lucie. This is important as this is what will be affected by the baclofen.

Ailsa will need to ask both parents about Lucie's birth history and developmental history to date. This will include Lucie's developmental milestones: at what age was Lucie able to roll over, sit on her own and crawl? Is she able to take weight through her legs? Lucie may not be able to carry out these activities yet, but her parents may still be working towards them. Ailsa will also need to ask about Lucie's general welfare. Does Lucie sleep well? If not, her spasticity may be making her difficult to position and therefore contributing to sleep problems or discomfort, causing her to wake up. Is Lucie eating lumpy food? At 18 months of age a child should be able to chew in order to eat a variety of textured food; however, this is often delayed in children with complex needs. If feeding for Lucie is difficult, how do the parents manage and is Lucie gaining weight appropriately? Has Lucie had any chest infections recently? Recurrent chest infections may be a sign of poor swallowing function, which would need further investigation before making changes to medication.

Ailsa will also need to ask Lucie's parents about her epilepsy. She has confirmed when Lucie had her last seizure. This is important as seizures must be well controlled before prescribing baclofen in order to monitor the effect of the medication on the child. Ailsa will also need to establish what a daily routine involves for Lucie. What equipment does she use? Are there any difficulties with using these? Who else is involved with caring for Lucie? (This may include different professionals or other family members or friends.)

Throughout the discussion with the parents Ailsa will also be observing Lucie. This would include looking at how she is responding, how she is sitting/moving and how her parents interact with her. As a physiotherapist, Ailsa would also carry out a physical assessment. This would allow her to assess Lucie's muscle tone, joint ranges and her general movement abilities. Ailsa would watch Lucie's responses carefully during the assessment.

The complex needs of children with cerebral palsy make it more difficult to precisely assess age-related development, especially cognitive ability. Cognitive ability will be assessed over a period of time and awareness of Lucie's development, combined with the provision of appropriate communication aids may allow a child to be able to effectively express their own views. However, the ability to give consent depends on being deemed to have the mental capacity required to make an informed decision. For many children with cerebral palsy this may not be possible to assess effectively.

It is good practice to include all children in the discussion in a consultation where possible, ensuring that any information is presented at an appropriate level for that child. Understanding what is happening often helps with the child's compliance, as they are more likely to cooperate with their parents if they have greater understanding.

In the UK, children aged 16 and 17 are able to consent to having a medical examination or treatment. Children who are under 16 and who are, in the professional's opinion, able to fully understand what is involved in the examination or procedure, can also give valid consent. Ideally parents should be involved and the professional should ask the young person's permission to consult or discuss matters with their parent(s). However, if this is withheld, the request for confidentiality should be respected. In general parents cannot overrule a valid consent given by a competent young person. However, even in a child who has been deemed competent, if there is a risk of the child suffering grave and irreversible mental or physical harm by refusing treatment, those with parental responsibility can override their decision.

For children who do not fit into the two categories described above, consent must be obtained from someone holding parental responsibility, unless there is an emergency and they cannot be contacted. This includes all children who do not have the capacity to consent. The power to consent must be used to ensure the child or young person's best interests are paramount. When working with children it is the parents that give their consent based on the best interests for their child. Practitioners need to ensure that those involved with the children are in a position to give their consent by determining who has parental responsibility. In this case both parents have parental responsibility as they were married at the time of the child's conception and neither parent loses parental responsibility if they divorce. As such Ailsa will ideally have to gain agreement from both parties although consent only needs to be obtained from someone holding parental responsibility. Occasionally there is conflict between two parents and the practitioner would then need to identify whether the cause of any conflict was due to genuine concern for the child or whether the objection could have been generated as a result of the marital dispute. There is a reluctance to overrule strongly held views and the discussion regarding the benefits and risks to the child should aim to reach a consensus acceptable to both parents.

In this case, once started, baclofen needs to be increased gradually and then given on a regular basis. When Lucie stays with her dad, he must continue to give her the baclofen as prescribed because serious side-effects can occur on abrupt withdrawal (Paediatric Formulary Committee, 2009). So Ailsa needs to ensure that both parents agree to use baclofen for Lucie.

If the parents had never been married, the practitioner would need to establish who does have parental responsibility. The mother has automatic parental responsibility when the parents have never married. Since 2002 (Adoption and Children Act) an unmarried father who has his name on the birth certificate has parental responsibility, along with the mother from the point of registration. If the child is not registered jointly, the father can acquire parental responsibility by entering into an agreement with the mother and registering it with the Principal Registry of the family division of the High Court. He would also gain parental responsibility if he subsequently married the mother.

In this case, if both or either parent refused consent, it would be appropriate for Ailsa to respect their wishes and to document the discussion. It may also be that parents may have a different opinion if the subject is revisited at a later date with a different decision being reached. However, if the refusal to consent to treatment is deemed to have a significant risk or negative outcome for the child, it would be the responsibility of the practitioner to seek further advice, which may include initiation of safeguarding procedures. This would not be the case with Lucie, as her symptoms are felt to be mild to moderate. However, if the child had severe spasticity, refusal by the parents to try medication may be deemed a safeguarding issue.

Q3   How can Ailsa ensure that the parents understand the possible benefits or risks involved in starting to use baclofen for Lucie?

Baclofen works by inhibiting transmission at spinal level and also by depressing the central nervous system. The medication directly affects the child's physical state. Baclofen has the positive outcome of reducing spasticity, which in turn may make functional activities such as nappy changing or handling easier for the carers. However, baclofen may also make the child drowsy or very floppy, which may in turn make it more difficult to handle the child or for the child to function. The assessment of changing function is one of the tools used to monitor both the possible positive or negative outcomes for individual children. The information gathered from the history provides the practitioner and parents with a baseline against which changes can be monitored.

The possible benefits of using baclofen for Lucie are that she may be less stiff in her muscles, allowing her to be cared for more easily. This would make essential functional activities such as nappy changing easier and quicker for both Lucie and her parents. Lucie may also be more comfortable in her equipment. By making these activities easier Lucie and her parents would have more time for playing and interacting. Lucie may also be able to move around more easily. She may be in less discomfort which may also help her to settle at night and therefore increase the amount of sleep that both she and her parents are able to achieve.

The main risks for Lucie are that she becomes drowsy or that her muscles become very floppy, making it more difficult for her to function. These side-effects of sedation and muscle hypotonia are avoided by increasing the dose slowly.

Baclofen has the potential to make life easier for Lucie and her parents but also has the potential to increase her difficulties. Ailsa will share with Lucie's parents what she feels would be the expected effects of the use of baclofen for Lucie. This should include what may improve for Lucie and also what to look out for regarding side-effects.

If it is shown that the benefits of using the medicine do not outweigh the risks, the effects can be reversed by discontinuing the baclofen gradually with dose reduction over a period of 1–2 weeks.

As both of Lucie's parents are involved in looking after her and responding to her needs, both need to be fully informed. Following the assessment, Ailsa should discuss with both parents the pros and cons of using baclofen and any other possible alternatives. Ultimately the decision to prescribe will be a shared one.

Q4   How could Ailsa involve Lucie's parents in monitoring her response to treatment?

As Lucie's parents are the ones who see her on a daily basis and know her best, they are the most appropriate people to monitor her response to treatment. Ailsa may identify specific functional activities that were presenting as a parental concern and ask them to monitor any changes. For example, the problem may have been that Lucie's legs were very stiff and it was difficult to open her legs in order to be able to clean her effectively during a nappy change. Ailsa will need to ask if this has become any easier following the treatment. She will also want to know if Lucie becomes more drowsy than usual. Both parents know what her usual state is and can therefore report any changes to Ailsa.

Ailsa may gain different information from Lucie's dad as he may notice changes from week to week as he sees her alternate weekends. Sometimes it is difficult to appreciate subtle changes when you are with a child all the time, but there may be changes over a two-week period. By putting all the information together from both parents, Ailsa will be able to build up a good picture of how Lucie is responding to treatment.

Scenario conclusion

Ailsa's assessment of Lucie, together with information from previous reports, meant she identified that Lucie's muscle tone had increased. In the consultation, Ailsa explained to both parents why it was that she felt that Lucie would benefit from having a trial period on an antispasmodic medicine. In order to gain consent from both parents, it was important that Ailsa addressed each of their concerns individually. A number of medicines were considered and ultimately both parents decided that a trial of baclofen would be appropriate.

Both parents gave consent to try baclofen and to monitor the effects closely. Ailsa started Lucie on the dose of 1 mg/kg daily (12 mg daily in three divided doses) with the aim of gradually increasing the dose to 2 mg/kg daily (24 mg daily in three divided doses) for maintenance. The parents were warned not to stop baclofen abruptly and to contact Ailsa if there were any concerns.

Initially there appeared to be no change for Lucie, but four weeks later her mum reported that she was finding it easier to change Lucie's nappy. Lucie remained alert and became more relaxed when in her equipment, which enabled her to begin to develop new skills.

Prescribing pitfalls

- Don't treat the child in isolation. When working with children, practitioners must work closely with parents to identify the best interests for each individual child.
- Parents know their children best. If they say something is wrong or different, believe them and investigate.
- Failure to take a good history as a baseline will make assessment to treatment very difficult.
- If you don't have parental consent and compliance, it is unlikely the medicine will be given/be effective.

Top tips

- Remember that it is a child you are prescribing for. Adjust the dosages according to the child's age and weight. And keep revisiting these.
- If a child is already taking medications, it is vital that potential interactions are examined. For example a different H_2-antagonist,

cimetidine, inhibits the metabolism of phenytoin but ranitidine does not. (Cimetidine has not been included in the 2009 *BNF for Children*; Paediatric Formulary Committee, 2009.)

- The prescriber always has a responsibility to act in the child's best interest.
- Consent can only be given by those who have parental responsibility for that child.
- Good communication with all parties involved is essential.

References

Paediatric Formulary Committee (2009) *BNF for Children*. London: BMJ Publishing Group, RPS Publishing, and RCPCH Publications.

Rosenbaum P, Paneth N, Leviton A, Goldstein M, Bax M (2007). A report: The definition and classification of cerebral palsy. April 2006. *Developmental Medicine and Child Neurology Supplement* 109: 8–14.

Further reading/websites of interest

Adoption and Children Act 2002. Chapter 38. www.opsi.gov.uk/acts/acts2002/ukpga_20020038_en_1

CMP Online Project (2010) Clinical management plans online. www.cmponline.info/

Department of Health (2009) Reference guide to consent for examination or treatment, 2nd edn. Consent key documents. www.dh.gov.uk/en/Publichealth/Scientificdevelopmentgeneticsandbioethics/Consent/Consentgeneralinformation/DH_119 [Accessed July 2009].

Department of Health (2010) Supplementary prescribing. http://webarchive.nationalarchives.gov.uk/+/www.dh.gov.uk/en/Healthcare/Medicinespharmacyandindustry/Prescriptions/TheNon-MedicalPrescribingProgramme/Supplementaryprescribing/index.htm [Accessed June 2010].

Nursing and Midwifery Council (2009) Advice sheet: Clinical management plans. www.nmc-uk.org/Nurses-and-midwives/Advice-by-topic/A/Advice/Clinical-Management-Plans-CMP/ [Accessed June 2010].

Paediatric Formulary Committee (2009) *BNF for Children*. http://bnfc.org

The Children Act 1989. Chapter 41. www.opsi.gov.uk/acts/acts1989/ukpga_19890041_en_1

The Children Act 2004. Chapter 31. www.opsi.gov.uk/acts/acts2004/ukpga_20040031_en_1

Mind map

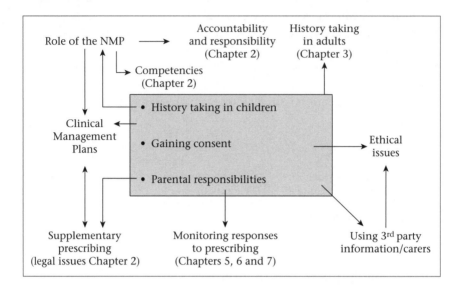

5

Prioritising in polypharmacy

Mike Jenkinson

Learning outcomes

After completing this chapter you will be able to:

- list considerations when prescribing in situations where altered pharmacokinetics/dynamics are likely (e.g. in renal failure, where there is polypharmacy or with medicines that undergo metabolic interactions);
- describe common outpatient medicine safety issues and suggest ways in which these problems may be prevented or addressed;
- understand how an experienced prescriber approaches prioritisation in a complex case.

Introduction

The issues around dosing are some of the most complex and important in therapeutics, because they require the prescriber to integrate individual patient characteristics with final delivery of a medicine. The medicine has usually been chosen from several possibilities that could produce a desired outcome. Getting the dose wrong will almost certainly impair that desired outcome. Too little medicine can be clinically ineffective, and too much can cause harm.

This chapter includes a complex case in an older patient. The reflective questions go into considerable detail in terms of the pharmacology underpinning this case. Don't be put off by this; we are really trying to illustrate the thinking a prescriber should undertake when considering prescribing decisions in a polypharmacy situation.

Prescriber

Martin Jolly joined The Larches Medical Centre 12 months ago as a new partner. He had previously worked for 5 years as a salaried general practitioner (GP) in another practice. Today, Thursday, he is assigned to deal with emergency home visits.

Patient background

John Williams is a 78-year-old man with a complex past medical history that includes type 2 diabetes, atrial fibrillation and heart failure after a myocardial infarction. His daughter visited him and his wife 3 days ago and today (2 days late) has phoned the surgery asking for a home visit. The daughter says Mr Williams has become more muddled, has a hacking cough and has badly swollen ankles. She reports that Mr Williams will 'under no circumstances go to hospital'. She tells the receptionist that the heart failure nurse had visited her father earlier in the week and had taken some blood and increased her father's water tablets.

Summary sheet with background information

Name: John Williams
DOB: 30/5/*seventy-eight years ago*
Occupation: Retired council administrator. Ex army major
Allergies: Allergic to penicillin (severe)

Past medical history

Hypertension for 18 years
Type 2 Diabetes mellitus *14 years ago*
Myocardial infarction and CABG *12 years ago*
Atrial fibrillation *10 years ago*
TIA *8 years ago*
Heart failure admission *6 years ago*
Gout *5 years ago*
TURP and NSTEMI *11 months ago*

$\longrightarrow$

Current medication

Atenolol 50 mg one in the morning
Digoxin 125 micrograms one in the morning
Warfarin 3 mg daily
Simvastatin 40 mg at night
Perindopril 2 mg daily
Spironolactone 25 mg in the morning
Furosemide 60 mg in the morning (increased from 40 mg in the
    morning *2 days ago*)
Tabphyn MR (tamsulosin) 400 micrograms at night
Avandamet (rosiglitazone/metformin) 2 mg/1 g twice a day
Colchicine 500 micrograms. Every 6 hours for 3 days for attack of
    gout and then leave off for 2 days

Disease monitoring (from previous day)

Hb: 12.2 g/dL (13–18)
WBC: 7×10^9/L (4–11)
Platelets: 246×10^9/L (150–400)
INR: 3.5
Sodium: 145 mmol/L (136–145)
Potassium: 5.9 mmol/L (3.5–5.1)
Creatinine: 246 micromol/L (64–104)
eGFR (MDRD estimate): 58 mL/min/1.73 m^2
CRP: 12 (0–10)
Capillary glucose (BM stix): 4.5 mmol/L
Temperature: 36.3°C
Pulse: 52 irregular
Blood pressure: 109/78 mmHg
Creps lung bases
++ Ankle oedema

Social history

Lives with wife in seaside flat chosen 13 years ago
Stopped smoking 12 years ago
Drinks red wine most evenings
Daughter lives 80 miles away, son overseas

Scenario

Martin consults Mr William's practice record and discovers that he has not seen a practice GP for 12 months. The heart failure nurse has been visiting regularly and yesterday requested a review for Mr Williams as his blood tests have deteriorated.

There is a comment from Martin's predecessor that implies Mr Williams complies with his medications well, although his aversion to hospital is documented. The last time Mr Williams saw a hospital doctor was in a consultant's clinic nine months ago. He was seen by a junior doctor in outpatients following transurethral resection of the prostate (TURP). The TURP was considered to be successful, although complicated by a non-ST elevation myocardial infarction (NSTEMI). The discharge summary at that time indicted 'heart follow-up' by the heart failure nurse. The junior hospital doctor had commented in the clinic letter that Mr Williams' heart failure was 'well controlled' and 'digoxin level is normal'. His creatinine was 114 micromol/L with the laboratory reporting an eGFR (MDRD estimate) of $54 \, mL/min/1.73 \, m^2$. After this Mr Williams did not attend appointments offered to him.

Martin phones Mr Williams and tries to persuade him to be admitted to hospital, but this meets with a definite refusal. He also asks for a home visit, to which Martin agrees. At the visit, Martin finds Mr Williams slightly confused but adamant that he will not accept hospitalisation. His wife confirms that he has become very 'pig headed' on the issue of admission to hospital. Last time he was in hospital the person in the next bed was noisy all night and actually tried to get into Mr Williams' bed, resulting in 'fisticuffs'. Mrs Williams says her husband has not been eating well for several weeks. This seemed to follow an attack of gout. He had to stop his colchicine when he started vomiting and had diarrhoea. The gout (and GI symptoms) subsequently resolved. He has been getting increasingly short of breath and has had to sleep in a recliner chair for two months.

Martin examines Mr Williams. He has quite marked ankle swelling, up to distal thigh. He has no focal consolidation on chest examination, although there are crepitations at both bases without any dullness. He is afebrile with pulse of 52 irregular and blood pressure is 109/78 mmHg. There is no bladder to percussion or new focal neurology.

Reflective questions

1   What general considerations are there when prescribing for older people?
2   What changes could Martin make to Mr Williams' medication immediately that might make him feel better?

3   What possible changes to Mr Williams' medications might Martin plan to make over the next week or two as matters hopefully stabilise?

Q1   What general considerations are there when prescribing for older people?

The use of medicines in older people is higher than in younger people. The National Service Framework for Older People suggests that four in five people over 75 take at least one prescribed medicine, with 36% taking four or more medicines (Department of Health, 2001). The increased incidence of interactions and adverse drug reactions (ADRs) that present as a result of this polypharmacy are a challenge for both prescriber and patient alike. Pharmacokinetic changes as a result of ageing can have profound effects, especially where clearance is affected. Dose alterations to accommodate age and disease-related renal failure need to be instituted and reviewed regularly. It can be difficult in older people to distinguish between ADRs and progression of the original disease. ADRs can induce non-specific symptoms such as confusion, dizziness (leading to a fall) or constipation. Frequently these go underreported by patients and undertreated by prescribers, who mistake ADRs for 'part of old age'. Similarly, normal manifestations of old age may be treated inappropriately. The role of prophylactic medication also has to be considered. A 92-year-old man should not be told to endure gastrointestinal symptoms because he is taking a statin that induced them.

Mr Williams presents a polypharmacy challenge. While there is the possibility that he has an undiagnosed condition that would explain his worsening renal failure, medicine toxicity alone could be playing the predominant role. Mr Williams' recent episode of colchicine-related vomiting and diarrhoea, coupled with his now low blood pressure, should make Martin suspicious. In other words, the renal failure could have started as mainly pre-renal, principally due to the dehydration. However, the accumulation of medicines excreted by the kidney could have led to renal toxicity themselves.

The *British National Formulary* (BNF) defines an eGFR (estimated glomerular filtration rate) between 30 and 59 mL/min/1.73 m^2 as moderate renal failure (Joint Formulary Committee, 2010). Medicine choices and dosing should reflect this. Martin would need to take into consideration the fact that published information on the effects of renal impairment on medicine elimination is usually stated in terms of creatinine clearance. The SPC (Summary of Product Characteristics, the manufacturer's description of a licensed medicine's properties) for a medicine will usually refer to creatinine clearance and even creatinine levels (for historic reasons) rather than eGFR. Prescribers need to remember that creatinine clearance is approximately equivalent to absolute GFR, but that the two measures of renal function, eGFR and creatinine clearance, are not interchangeable. An individual's absolute GFR can be calculated from the eGFR as follows:

$$GFR_{absolute} = eGFR \times (individual's\ body\ surface\ area/1.73)$$

If an estimation is being made of renal function using a serum creatinine value, the Cockcroft and Gault equation is used (see BNF, Joint Formulary Committee, 2010). However, this requires knowledge of not only the weight of the individual, but also their height. While the equation itself only includes weight, this is only appropriate if that individual's weight falls within the normal body weight range for a person of that age. If they fall outside the normal range, Cockcroft and Gault would be considered less reliable. In a frail elderly person, the Cockcroft and Gault estimated creatinine clearance would overestimate clearance and the result would need to be corrected downwards to provide a cut-off for safe use of the medicine.

It is important for Martin to establish rapport with Mr Williams and his family and involve him as a partner in all decisions relating to his care. In order to do this, Martin has to first address his own feelings. The patient has refused advice that Martin sees as being in Mr Williams' best interests. Mr Williams will need considerable time and resources devoted to him, which would be easier to coordinate in hospital. Martin would be ill-advised to labour the point that Mr Williams has rejected his advice, but he should mention (and document that he has done so) that it is possible that the condition has reached a potentially life-threatening stage which would be much easier to assess and treat in hospital.

However, if Mr Williams is fully informed of the situation, but still refuses admission, Martin must respect his decisions as far as possible. There is potential that coordination, with continuity of care between Martin and the heart failure nurse, will actually result in a good outcome for Mr Williams. If Mr Williams' trust is regained, he may feel happy to accept a hospital referral in the near future.

Good history taking is also dependent on establishing a good rapport with the patient and the carer. Mr Williams is somewhat confused and Martin will need to piece together what has been happening from a number of sources of information. Whenever medicine toxicity is possible, a careful and directed history is needed, to identify any change in a medication or other factors shortly before the symptoms started. Mr Williams has had an increase in his diuretic dose in the last few days which has already potentially worsened the pre-renal element of his renal failure. It should also be borne in mind that minor insult, such as the vomiting and diarrhoea due to colchicine, might trigger dehydration and further phys-iological decompensation. Mrs Williams has mentioned this to Martin, but many patients on colchicine take these side-effects for granted and in fact use them as an indicator of when they must stop the medicine during an acute attack. Some patients might not even mention the episode of diar-rhoea and sickness and so a vital 'clue' may not have been picked up without specific questioning.

Q2   What changes could Martin make to Mr Williams' medication immediately that might make him feel better?

The first key point when dealing with a complex polypharmacy situation is to consider which medicines are contributing to any immediate life-threatening toxicity. Here, the real risk is cardiac arrhythmia (but in another context, it could be seizures, respiratory or cardiac depression). Martin needs to deal with the high potassium. Mr Williams' potassium is bordering a potentially toxic level and might have reached a toxic level in the day that has passed since his blood test.

The acute treatment and frequent monitoring of electrolytes required in life-threatening hyperkalaemia are not practical in the community. For example, an urgent ultrasound to exclude hydronephrosis (blockage of the urinary tract) would be carried out if Mr Williams were an inpatient. However, the potassium level is not so high that it needs treatment with insulin/glucose infusion and calcium intravenously, which could only be carried out in hospital, so home treatment is still possible. *Immediate change number 1* is to stop the potassium-sparing diuretic spirinolactone and the ACE inhibitor perindopril, both of which cause hyperkalaemia, while maintaining (or even slightly increasing) the furosemide. This will almost certainly deal with the potassium situation in a few days.

Although Martin almost certainly would be familiar with the use of ion-exchange resins such as calcium resonium, he is perhaps best advised not to use them here. There could be a delay in filling the script and their use requires frequent electrolyte monitoring in this situation. Martin should consider that with rapidly recovering kidney function, life-threatening hypokalaemia, especially in a patient on digoxin, can develop with only a few doses.

Heart failure decompensation is unlikely in the short term, as spir-onolactone will continue its actions on the angiotensin system for several days and there are other reasons outlined below why there is likely to be a fairly large diuresis in the next few days. It should be realised that paradox-ically the high potassium is cardioprotective to a degree.

Cardioprotection is desirable here because the renal failure (and the anorexia with confusion) indicates we have a situation of almost certain digoxin toxicity. Martin does not need blood levels or even an ECG to suspect this and act. Digoxin has a narrow therapeutic index and he knows the level was in the normal therapeutic range (for atrial fibrillation) reported by the laboratory nine months ago. As digoxin is renally secreted and renal function has decreased, toxicity has ensued. Martin must stop the digoxin (*immediate change number 2*). He will no doubt arrange to check the digoxin level as soon as possible and this might give an idea as to when to recommence the digoxin in due course. The long half-life of the medicine might easily necessitate a wait of a week or more.

Once Martin has established which medicines are contributing to the immediate life-threatening toxicity and has stopped those, he needs to address the second key point, which is to ask if are there any medicines in this situation that are contraindicated or that can be stopped with low likelihood of immediate harm. One suggestion here is to assume the medicines you know less well will need more effort to understand than those you know well. However, if the medicine is used more rarely for a common condition it might be because it is relatively ineffective.

Mr Williams is on Avandamet, which may well be because of a historic decision by another doctor as it was more popular in the past. If Martin does not use this medicine in his practice, he should look it up in the BNF. It is a rosiglitazone/metformin combination and has been marketed in three different dose combinations. Although combination products are more convenient in stable patients and might aid compliance, a potential downside is the difficulty of dose adjustment in unstable patients. Rosiglitazone is contraindicated in patients with a history of heart failure and has a specific recommendation that it should be used with caution in severe renal failure.

While long-term studies have shown that metformin improves cardiovascular outcome in diabetes, there is less convincing evidence of such benefit from rosiglitazone, despite its effect on glycaemic control. This may be due to other medicine-specific properties. The long-term mortality and morbidity data for rosiglitazone and pioglitazone currently favour pioglitazone. Martin should stop the rosiglitazone by stopping the Avandamet (*immediate change number 3*). As glitazones seem to block some of the action of loop diuretics, this might also help promote diuresis.

Metformin is contraindicated in renal failure. Confidence has grown in using it in patients with creatinine levels up to about 130 micromol/L because of its beneficial effects on mortality. However, the marketing authorisation contraindicates it in even mild renal failure (creatinine clearance <60 mL/min). This is because an analogue no longer marketed had a risk of lactic acidosis. The specific risk of lactic acidosis with metformin is controversial. The BNF recommends at least six monthly renal monitoring. It is not important to obtain good blood sugar control in the short term (although fair control is likely for some time as the medicines will take days to clear from the system). Indeed, use of insulin is unlikely to be necessary. Perhaps in a few weeks, if necessary, a diabetic specialist might recommend that Mr Williams goes back on metformin alone if his renal function recovers.

An underlying problem in Mr Williams' history for the last nine months has been mild renal failure. The unstated problem now is that his current blood pressure is unexpectedly low for a man with a past history of hypertension. It is possible that the choice of a renally secreted beta-blocker with a longish half-life (atenolol) rather than a predominantly hepatically metabolised beta-blocker could have played a role in the development of his renal failure if accumulation has occurred. The atenolol, with its water solubility and renal secretion is not an ideal beta-blocker to use in renal failure and it has a weaker evidence base for effectiveness in heart failure. It is a bad idea, however, to suddenly stop beta-blockers in patients with potentially unstable ischaemic heart disease. The evidence base suggests there are more vascular events after suddenly stopping beta-blockers, anti-platelet agents and statins. Martin should consider changing atenolol to a low dose of bisoprolol, a beta-blocker with a good evidence base in treating heart failure. The others that fall into this category, carvedilol and nebivolol, have renal failure cautions. Atenolol 50 mg is approximately equivalent to bisoprolol 5 mg (hint – look at the range of recommended doses for each medicine in the BNF when you substitute in a class of medicines). So, stopping the atenolol 50 mg and substituting bisoprolol 2.5 mg daily (*immediate change number 4*) would be a good choice for Mr Williams.

As tamsulosin is predominantly hepatically metabolised it is a suitable alpha-blocker in mild to moderate renal failure. If it is stopped, it will certainly help renal perfusion by increasing the blood pressure. It probably should be withheld until at least the blood pressure is above 120 systolic and in due course either finasteride or dutasteride offered to control prostatic symptoms if they should occur. Indeed it could have been removed (as a therapeutic trial) after the successful TURP, so Martin would be recommended to stop the tamsulosin now and re-evaluate (*immediate change number 5*). There have been rare reports of confusion with alpha-blockers and they do not increase survival in heart failure.

There have been multiple changes in medications and many of the medicines being started and stopped modify warfarin metabolism, meaning INR control may not be easy. In the context of a high but acceptable INR and an acute illness an experienced hospital doctor would reduce the warfarin dose by about 25%, knowing not to expect an effect on the INR for up to 3 days. This is based on the fact that mild under-anticoagulation is safer than over-anticoagulation. The target is still an INR around 2.5. The guidance is to repeat the INR a week after a change in therapy, as the current figure is therapeutic. This is an example of where prescribers are expected to deviate from guidelines in the patient's interest and of course document the reasons. In this case, the complexity of the medication changes and Mr Williams' refusal to go to hospital means that it is best to err on the side of caution. Mr Williams will need his potassium and creatinine checked within 24 hours of Martin's visit and again a few days after this. The INR can be done at the same time. Martin could immediately reduce the warfarin to 2 mg daily. Once Mr Williams' medication regimen is stable, Martin will be advised, particularly if the slight confusion did not resolve completely, to reconsider anticoagulation.

Q3   What possible changes to Mr Williams' medications might Martin plan to make over the next week or two as matters hopefully stabilise?

Martin has to consider the restart of Mr Williams' digoxin (*longer term prescribing consideration number 1*). If he uses digoxin levels to help him, he would be advised to consider two issues. The first is that survival in male patients in heart failure is maximised with digoxin levels in the range 0.5 to 0.9 ng/mL. Many laboratories quote so called 'therapeutic' ranges as up to 2 ng/mL or more as these are the normal therapeutic ranges to control resting heart rate in atrial fibrillation. Usual treatment of atrial fibrillation has changed in the last 20 years to use a rate-controlling medicine such as a beta-blocker (possibly also selected for its benefit in heart failure) and so modern optimal treatment levels of digoxin are often at the lower limits of the therapeutic range reported by a laboratory. The second issue for consideration in relation to digoxin is that toxicity is also a function of cations such as potassium and magnesium. It is quite possible to have digoxin concentrations in the higher 'therapeutic' range and manifest digoxin toxicity with serum potassium levels around 3.0 mmol/L. As Mr Williams will be managed on potassium (and magnesium)-sparing diuretics in the future, it would be a good idea for Martin to aim for a relatively low digoxin concentration, even if it does not obtain adequate resting heart rate control without help by another medicine. On restarting digoxin, Martin will use a dose of no more than 62.5 micrograms.

Having reduced the warfarin initially, Martin needs to revisit the question of anticoagulation for Mr Williams (*longer term prescribing consideration number 2*). An unstable INR is a good reason to consider stopping anticoagulation, as it directly correlates with bleeding risk and issues such as confusion or the potential for further increase in red wine ingestion would make Martin concerned. The fact that presently there are no proven alternatives to anticoagulation in atrial fibrillation stroke prevention, should not prevent Martin from stopping the warfarin. With a history of ischaemic heart disease, Mr Williams should be started on antiplatelet therapy. Mr Williams' recently active gout means that low-dose aspirin is not suitable. The significant changes in urate handling in elderly patients with low-dose aspirin (75 mg) are well described, and are responsible for increased morbidity in those with renal failure. Clopidrogel should therefore be considered for secondary prevention of ischaemic heart disease. The prevention of stroke is no longer the most important factor in the choice of medicine. The reason is that when Mr Williams had his NSTEMI 11 months ago while on warfarin, he was not put on an antiplatelet agent. It is known that warfarin is equivalent in total morbidity/mortality clinical outcomes to antiplatelet agents. Combination therapy has no advantages in total morbidity/mortality in the very old. Consensus guidelines have recently been published recommending that in anticoagulated patients presenting with acute coronary syndrome anticoagulation can be combined with antiplatelet treatment at the time of highest risk of a coronary event, reverting to anticoagulation alone when this risk is past. However, once warfarin is removed from the equation, the recent NSTEMI is the most important issue affecting his morbidity/mortality risk, and so an antiplatelet agent is likely to be beneficial.

The simvastatin can be continued. There could be an argument for brief dose reduction as severe renal failure increases the risk of side-effects such as rhabdomyolysis. The BNF states that doses higher than 10 mg should not be used if eGFR is $<30 \, mL/minute/1.73 \, m^2$.

Treatment of Mr Williams' gout will need Martin's long-term consideration (*longer term prescribing consideration number 3*). Colchicine may no longer be considered after its possible involvement in this incident. Any NSAID such as diclofenac, naproxen or indometacin would be ruled out as they worsen renal and heart failure. There is trial evidence to back-up the clinical observation that a short course of moderate-dose prednisolone is effective in acute gout (Janssens *et al.*, 2008). This took over 50 years to prove in a randomised controlled trial. Two generations of doctors have been biased against steroids in gout after work in the 1950s in which steroids given continuously to control gout resulted in poor outcomes.

Scenario conclusion

Martin is pleased when Mr William's renal condition gradually improves over the next few weeks, through care from both himself and the heart failure nurse. Martin speaks to the local elderly specialist care physician and, under his watchful eye, Martin cautiously reintroduces renin–

angiotensin blockade to treat the heart failure. This involves monitoring electrolytes initially weekly. Because of Mr Williams' gout Martin starts him on losartan, as it has urisuric effects not shared with any other angiotensin II blocker (or ACE inhibitor). The downside is that it has been shown to be less effective in heart failure and may accumulate in severe renal impairment. However, Martin and the heart failure nurse are regular visitors at the Williams' household and Martin feels he will be ready to act to any change in Mr Williams' condition.

Prescribing pitfalls

- Avoid adopting a 'one size fits everyone' approach (e.g. low-dose aspirin for all). Prescribers must consider patient-specific factors such as potential for gout or risk of bleeding.
- Do not automatically assume combination products are the best choice. They may have marketable attractions like compliance, but have potential safety issues and challenges in dose adjustment.
- Do not assume all medicines in a class are the same. For example, losartan is the only urisuric sartan.
- Avoid prioritising treatment of the wrong condition in patients with complex pathology just because a treatment is available.
- The BNF lists of cautions and side-effects are a very useful aide-memoire in tailoring medicine therapy to individual patients. The BNF is weaker, however, in guiding prescribers to the best choice of medicine within a medicine class.

Top tips

- Beware of potential for drug interactions. Only a few medicines are the common culprits – know these medicines well and assume there will be a medicine interaction until proven otherwise.
- Know common medicines for common conditions – these should be part of your P drug list (see Chapter 1). However, a prescriber who only knows one medicine from a class well, when there are several on the market, is probably not optimising therapy in complex patients. Medicines in the same class have different properties. Learning the class properties may help the differences stand out.
- Polypharmacy increases the chances of interaction both with other medicines and with other pathologies.
- Adjust doses for renal and hepatic failure. It is especially important to monitor renal function carefully as people get older.

- Medicine side-effects may aggravate a pre-existing condition and need to be considered when selecting a medicine. Patient-specific information must also be factored in to maximise safe and effective medicine taking.
- Serum monitoring of a medicine to determine optimal treatment can be very useful where there is a good evidence base, as in digoxin in heart failure.
- Even short courses of a medicine can cause significant problems, but this is more likely with a high pre-existing (medicine) load.

References

Department of Health (2001) *National Service Framework for Older People*. London: Department of Health.

Janssens HJE, Janssen M, van de Lisonk EH, van Riel PLCM and van Weel C (2008). Use of oral prednisolone or naproxen for the treatment of gout arthritis: a double-blind, randomised equivalence trial. *Lancet* 371: 1854–1860.

Joint Formulary Committee (2010) *BNF: British National Formulary 60*. London: British Medical Association and Royal Pharmaceutical Society of Great Britain, October.

Further reading/websites of interest

The BNF has a good section on prescribing in renal failure generally. From BNF 59 onwards the information about prescribing in renal failure for each individual drug is included in the monograph for the drug, rather than in a single appendix.

For understanding the strengths and weakness and context of the MDRD formula for GFR, see www.renal.org/eGFR/eguide.html.

For some of the drug interactions that produce real problems see www.mhra.gov.uk/Publications/Safetyguidance/DrugSafetyUpdate/index.htm e.g. Statins: interactions, and updated advice. Drug Safety Update: January 2008; 1(6):2.

If the information on a medicine in the BNF is insufficient in a particular patient situation a useful source of information is the SPC (Summary of Product Characteristics) for a medicine. For most POM (Prescription Only Medicines) or P (Pharmacy Only Medicines) medications these are available at the electronic Medicines Compendium (eMC) website http://emc.medicines.org.uk.

It is important to understand that the same clinical evidence on medicines can be interpreted differently by different prescribers and medical subcultures. For example the standard dose regimen of colchicine recommended in the USA (and American text books) historically is much higher than that in recent British practice. The evidence for best dosing is at www.fda.gov/Drugs/DrugSafety/PostmarketDrugSafetyInformationforPatients andProviders/DrugSafetyInformationforHeathcareProfessionals/ucm174315.htm (Information for Healthcare Professionals: New Safety Information for Colchicine marketed as Colcrys. FDA ALERT [07/30/2009]).

There are multiple sources of information on small print medicine issues but a Medline/PubMed (www.ncbi.nlm.nih.gov/sites/entrez)/NHS evidence (www.evidence.nhs.uk/) search tends to be quite effective.

For the small-print issue of losartan and gout the following reference has the advantage that it is recent and the whole article is free to access in a peer-reviewed journal. Iwanaga T, Sato M, Maeda T, Ogihara T, Tamai I (2007) Concentration-dependent mode of interaction of angiotensin II receptor blockers with uric acid transporter. *Journal of Pharmacology and Experimental Therapeutics* 320: 211–217.

The European Society of Cardiology consensus guidelines on combined antiplatelet and anticoagulation therapy in established atrial fibrillation is free to access and deals comprehensively with a difficult area. Lip GY, Huber K, Andreotti F, *et al.* (2010) Management of antithrombotic therapy in atrial fibrillation patients presenting with acute coronary syndrome and/or undergoing percutaneous coronary intervention/stenting. *Thrombosis and Haemostasis* 103: 13–28.

Mind map

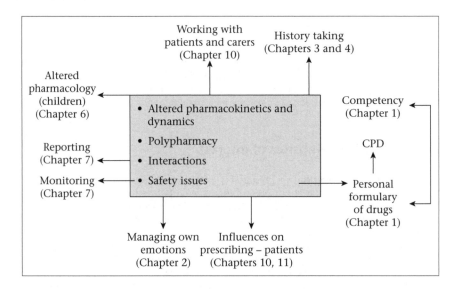

6

Practical prescribing in paediatrics

Elizabeth Worthing

Learning outcomes

After completing this chapter you will be able to:

- identify information sources that guide paediatric prescribing practice and outline their limitations;
- review the different methods for calculating drug dosing in children, apply good prescription writing etiquette and recognise potential pitfalls in practice;
- describe the complexities of medicine administration in children, appreciate that lack of appropriate formulations may compromise optimal outcomes and navigate the use of unlicensed medicines.

Introduction

Children can present with a wide spectrum of conditions and disease states, and their individual personalities and family relationships will be equally varied. Each situation is unique, making paediatric prescribing practice both broad and stretching. The youngest patient may be a premature baby of 23 weeks gestation, and the oldest 16 years old, with some specialist clinics planning to continue treatment up to 25 years old. This diverse group will undergo an extensive range of developmental changes over this period of their life.

A lack of clinical trials in children has resulted in patchy knowledge of paediatric drug handling and inadequate provision of paediatric formulations. There is an estimated current use of unlicensed/off-label medicines in approximately 10% of paediatric primary care and 90% of specialist neonatal practice. Recent legislation aims to stimulate new research, expand the range and availability of paediatric medicines, and facilitate communication between professionals, carers, children and adolescents, thus bridging the gap between clinical obligations and current resources.

This chapter demonstrates that when prescribing for children, it is important to have a good understanding of underpinning pharmacology, but that practical issues may often hold the key to successful treatment.

Prescriber

Ellen Miller is a paediatric pharmacist with background experience of working overseas in tertiary care. She is now based in a district general hospital and grapples with the practicalities of providing secondary care services to the paediatric and neonatal units. The average length of hospital stay for children in the paediatric wards is 16–18 hours, and much of this admission time is spent without parental attendance. This brings priority setting and communication challenges to her practice.

Patient background

The patient in this case is Lucie Bothy, who also featured in Chapter 4. In this chapter we see how another healthcare professional prescriber approaches aspects of her care. It is three months later and Lucie is now aged 21 months.

Summary sheet with background information

Name: Lucie Bothy
Age: 21 *months*
Current weight: 12 kg
Current height: 81 cm

Past medical history

Born at 28 weeks gestation
Ventilated for six weeks on SCBU
Discharged home at 38 weeks still requiring oxygen

$\longrightarrow$

Gastro-oesophageal reflux disorder (GORD) diagnosed age six months – managed with ranitidine

Baclofen started aged 18 months to help with spasticity

Current medication

Phenytoin 60 mg twice daily orally (5 mg/kg twice daily) for seizure control

Ranitidine 24 mg twice daily orally (2 mg/kg twice daily) for GORD

Baclofen 4 mg three times daily orally (1 mg/kg/day) for spasticity

Social history

Lucie is an only child

She lives with her mother and spends alternate weekends with her father

Her parents are divorced

Scenario

Following the introduction of baclofen, Lucie's parents both attended the next three-monthly outpatient appointment to review Lucie's progress and medicine management. Lucie's mother commented that the spasticity had initially improved, but she was again struggling with handling, and Lucie had frequent runny stools. Lucie's father said that the baclofen dosing was difficult and wondered if there was some simpler way to give the medicine.

Reflective questions

1 Before she starts to address Lucie's issues, where could Ellen find information sources for paediatric prescribing? How might different sources express children's dosing schedules?

2 As Ellen contemplates prescribing for Lucie, what are common slips to guard against when writing paediatric prescriptions?

3 What pharmacokinetic changes occur between the neonatal and early infant period, and what precautions should be taken in prescribing and administering Lucie's antiepileptic medicines?

4 At the three-monthly outpatient appointment it is evident that 'following the recommended dosing rate' has led to dosing difficulties for Lucie's father, and

using 'licensed products' has resulted in a problem of loose stools. How did this happen, what other problems could arise, and what are alternative prescribing approaches?

5   What prescribing issues may arise in the long-term management of Lucie's chronic condition?

Q1   Before she starts to address Lucie's issues, where could Ellen find information sources for paediatric prescribing?

Ellen would find two review articles 'Prescribing for children' from the National Prescribing Centre (2000), and 'Prescribing in children' from Patient UK (2010) helpful in summarising core prescribing principles. She should also read 'Making medicines safer for children – guidance for the use of unlicensed medicines in paediatric patients' (Tomlin *et al.*, 2009). This article presents case studies from the UK illustrating practice pitfalls encountered with unlicensed medicines.

Ellen should also check that she has up-to-date editions of respected prescribing texts. She may prefer to consult more than one reference, as this will give her a broad base for decision making. However, this may not always be possible due to time constraints, and some people find this approach confusing. The first reference for her current practice will be the *BNF for Children* (BNFc) (Paediatric Formulary Committee, 2010), which provides information across the full paediatric age range. She will also use the standard *British National Formulary* (BNF), which contains detailed adolescent dosing, but summarises information on younger ages (Joint Formulary Committee, 2010). Two other supporting British references include the *Neonatal Formulary* (Northern Neonatal Network, 2007) and the *Paediatric Formulary* (Guy's, St. Thomas' and Lewisham Hospitals, 2010). Both provide alphabetically arranged drug monographs, the former focusing on neonates and the latter with additional guidelines and protocols. Different prescribing approaches are supported by the *Pediatric Dosage Handbook* published in North America (Taketomo *et al.*, 2010). This incorporates pharmacokinetic data into each drug monograph, with an extensive appendix of laboratory values and clinical guidelines. Finally, *Drug Doses*, an abbreviated Australian text, summarises drug dosing in a pocket-sized booklet (Frank Shann Collective, 2008).

Q2   As Ellen contemplates prescribing for Lucie, what are common slips to guard against when writing paediatric prescriptions?

Prescription writing 'etiquette' is particularly pertinent in paediatric prescribing, and Ellen will find core practice principles are summarised in the introductory section in the BNFc. Prescribing via electronic programmes has the advantage of flagging up medicine interactions, but use of these systems is not trouble free. Choice of medicine is commonly selected by entering the first three letters of the medicine name into the computer, then choosing the required medicine and formulation from the displayed menu. All prescribers must guard against situations where a different medicine is punched in haste; for example, sal-meterol when sal-butamol is intended, or an inappropriate formulation, such as paracetamol injection for home use.

There are a variety of different methods used to express paediatric dosing schedules such as mg/kg/dose, mg/kg/day, mg/age, mg/m^2, mL/kg or mL/age. This variety requires that focused and careful attention must be given during the prescribing process to prevent misreading or misapplication of the dosing schedules with serious consequences. In general, fewer errors occur when regimens are calculated as mg/kg/dose, rather than by mg/kg/day divided by the frequency of administration. The latter calculation requires two mathematical steps, a multiplication followed by a division, and division processes attract a high error rate. In addition, this style of dosing schedule can result in overdosing if it is misread as mg/kg/*dose*, *multiplied* by the frequency. Dosing by age or weight banding has been introduced into some units to simplify and speed practice, but these calculations are inherently imprecise and they may be misinterpreted, or applied to children that do not have a normal weight for age. Dosing as mg/m^2 is the most precise method for children over three months, but this requires measurement of weight and height (length in children under 3 years), and this form of dosing information is available for a limited number of medicines only. Caution is required when using mL/kg or mL/age regimens, particularly when there are liquid formulations of varying strengths.

Good prescribing habits should always include a quick mental calculation to estimate the expected dose. This extra step acts as a safety check and will usually highlight if an error has been made with the use of calculators.

Q3   What pharmacokinetic changes occur between the neonatal and early infant period, and what precautions should be taken in prescribing and administering Lucie's antiepileptic medicines?

Lucie was delivered prematurely at 28 weeks gestation, and would therefore undergo significant maturation processes in the immediate days and weeks following birth (Costello, 2007; Kearns *et al.*, 2003) with attendant changes reflected in laboratory values (Verras and Greaves, 2005). Treatment for her neonatal seizures was initiated by the intravenous (IV) route, since oral absorption in neonates and young children is variable due to high gastric pH, erratic gastric emptying, reduced intestinal motility and immature secretion of biliary salts. Neonates also have a greater proportion of total body water with a larger volume of distribution than adults, and require higher loading doses.

When the phenytoin dose was to be loaded, Ellen would have discovered that the BNFc recommends an IV loading dose in neonates of 18 mg/kg, whereas the BNF lists a range of 15–20 mg/kg, and the *Neonatal Formulary* and *Paediatric Formulary* both give 20 mg/kg. Selecting a mid-range dose of 18 mg/kg would be good prescribing practice, as would be annotating the calculated dose with '18 mg/kg loading dose'. This provides a safety check for other professionals that review the prescription. Before this prescription was signed, an attentive second check should be undertaken. Choonara (1999) lists phenytoin as a 'high risk' medicine that can cause significant harm if a mistake is made; therefore a third self-check is warranted before the prescription is finally issued. When the consultant asked Ellen which dosing rate she had chosen for Lucie, she replied, 'eighteen milligrams per kilogram', and then added, 'one, eight'. This method ensured that the rate was communicated clearly, rather than mis-heard as 'eighty milligrams per kilogram'.

Although good control can be achieved with phenytoin, alternative drug choices such as lidocaine are of current interest. This product does not contain propylene glycol which is now recognised to be neurotoxic in neonates. In addition, as phenytoin injection has been formulated for adult use, it requires careful dilution for neonatal use. The *Neonatal Formulary* points out that overlooking the presence of medicine contained in the hub of a syringe can result in inaccurate dilution and inadvertent administration of three times the intended dose in neonates. Therefore Lucie's antiepileptic therapy, which used a concentrated solution of a medicine that has a narrow therapeutic window, must be carefully prescribed, measured, administered and monitored.

Enteral feeds interfere with the absorption of oral phenytoin (White and Bradnam, 2007) so changing Lucie's anticonvulsant therapy to the oral route would have been delayed until normal feeding was introduced and well established. Phenytoin oral dosing schedules vary with age to reflect pharmacokinetic changes. Neonates have low gastric acid secretion with impaired absorption, so initial dosing rates are higher than in infants. However, as metabolism increases, the dosing rate also increases, before stabilisation. Throughout these changes, Lucie's actual prescribed dose will need to steadily increase as her weight increases.

Well before discharge, Lucie's parents will be counselled on the purpose of all of her medicines, possible side-effects to look out for and how the medicines should be handled. Grießmann *et al.* (2007) have demonstrated that use of flat-bottomed spoons may deliver up to 219% of an intended dose, and commented that spoons or medicine cups with a narrow base area, or preferably, oral syringes have greater accuracy. Since small changes in phenytoin dosing result in big changes in effect, both of Lucie's parents should be asked to demonstrate correct use of an oral syringe.

Phenytoin suspension also contains sucrose as a sweetening agent, so chronic use puts Lucie at risk of developing dental caries. The chewable Infatabs™ also contain sucrose, whereas the capsules are sugar free. However, these solid dose forms do not have the precision and flexibility of dosage adjustment that is required for phenytoin dosing in a growing child. Lucie's parents should therefore be counselled additionally on the need to rinse Lucie's mouth after use of the suspension.

Q4   At the three-monthly outpatient appointment it is evident that 'following the recommended dosing rate' has led to dosing difficulties for Lucie's father, and using 'licensed products' has resulted in a problem of loose stools. How did this happen, what other problems could arise, and what are alternative prescribing approaches?

At the three-monthly outpatient appointment, Ellen reviews Lucie's prescribed schedule for baclofen (1 mg/kg/day divided into three doses), and calculates that each individual dose measures 3.66 mL. The practicality of measuring a dose of 3.66 mL means that Lucie was unlikely to receive the correct dose, so she decides to increase the dose to 4 mL per dose (i.e. 1.09 mg/kg daily). This situation can occur in paediatric prescribing where the 'correctly calculated' dose is not easily deliverable. A pragmatic approach needs to be taken. Lucie's father is pleased with the change and confesses to having rounded down the dose to make weekend dosing simpler!

Excipients are included in the formulation of the vast majority of medicines and this can be a significant issue in medicines use by children. Since the appearance of the loose stools coincided with the introduction of the baclofen, Ellen might suspect that this could have been precipitated by the excipient sorbitol, a 'sugar-free' sweetening agent which is contained in both the baclofen and ranitidine formulations, and in many other suspensions. Additional concerns in Lucie's case might include the presence of 7.5% alcohol in the licensed ranitidine syrup. Although little is known about the effects of chronic alcohol ingestion in children, the US Food and Drug Administration (FDA) have set a limit of <0.5% alcohol for children under the age of six (FDA, 1995). Alcohol-free formulations with limited shelf-lives are available as unlicensed 'specials' with legal responsibility resting with Ellen as prescriber and the procurement pharmacist, not the manufacturer. Ellen could reasonably decide to investigate whether a suitable ranitidine formulation is available, before changing GORD management to a proton pump inhibitor.

Lucie is also at risk for developing repeated chest infections, and will almost certainly require regular high-dose antibiotic treatment at some stage. This can precipitate loose stools as a side-effect, with additional irritation from a sore nappy area. This should be managed by intensive nappy hygiene, together with oral and topical antifungals if candidiasis is suspected. Dietary yogurt can be helpful. Emollients on their own have anti-inflammatory activity, whereas topical application of a mild cortico-steroid should be prescribed with care. When necessary, sparing application and brief duration are in order. Systemic absorption is a risk in infants, who have a higher ratio of body surface area to body weight than adults, greater hydration and perfusion, and reduced skin thickness. In addition, the nappy itself acts as an occlusive dressing. Confusion can arise in pre-scribing between the mild form of corticosteroid hydrocortisone acetate 1%, and the potent preparation hydrocortisone butyrate 0.1%. The latter can damage the skin structure in young children.

Although current UK practice favours the supply of liquid formula-tions to children, the World Health Organization supports extending the availability and range of paediatric solid oral formulations such as small dose tablets and capsules, with the potential benefits of reduced excipients, increased shelf-life, convenience of transport, and reduced haulage costs. Whatever choices are made, all medicine and formulation details, and rationale for choices should be clearly communicated between all practi-tioners in primary, secondary and tertiary areas to avoid unnecessarily capsizing Lucie's management at the next port of call.

Q5   What prescribing issues may arise in the long-term management of Lucie's chronic condition?

At some future stage Lucie may develop severe swallowing difficulties with a high risk of aspiration. This situation is managed by insertion of an enteral feeding tube and administration of feeds and medicines through the tube. Some medicines, such as phenytoin, may interact with the feeds, requiring separation of one or two hours between administration of the medicine and the feed. All medicines will require a flush before and after administration to ensure passage down the tube without risk of blockage. Good care of the tube and attention to the timing of administration is vital (White and Bradnam, 2007).

If feeding problems associated with Lucie's condition are resolved successfully, her lack of mobility potentially puts her at risk of becoming obese. Optimal growth rates based on breastfed infants have recently been redefined, and revised growth charts are available (see BNFc summary table). Although there are still gaps in our knowledge about pharmacokinetic medicine handling in obese children, because these children have a larger muscle and kidney mass than children of normal weight, their renal clearance may be greater. It will be important to monitor Lucie's weight and clinical response to her medicines closely.

Children with chronic conditions rapidly gain knowledge of their condition and become 'expert' patients. There are anecdotal stories of pre-school 4-year-old asthmatic children organising their own inhaler management in the absence of parental supervision. However, development of maturity may not keep pace with children's clinical knowledge, and this may cause tensions in various relationships as the child becomes older. Treatment failure is known to have occurred simply because a child did not like the colour of the tablets they received, and although alternatives were available, the child had never been consulted about choice. Although Lucie is totally dependent on adult carers, she will still have her own unique personality with her own set of 'likes' and 'dislikes'. Prescribers for children should be aware of these issues and review guidance on establishing and maintaining good communication with children and teenagers (Hummelinck and Pollock, 2007; Gray, 2008).

Prescribing pitfalls

- Avoid guessing the child's dose; refer to a reputable reference.
- Don't be afraid to question a colleague's prescribing decision if you have any concerns. Even consultants make mistakes – we are all human!
- Don't fail to cap adolescent doses at adult levels; remember that you are not prescribing for a baby elephant!
- Don't forget that neonatal and paediatric laboratory values may be different from those for adults.
- Never, never rush when prescribing a 'high-risk' medicine – the risk is too high!

Top tips

- Read dosing references carefully and select the regimen that is the most appropriate.
- Listen first – then adjust the dosing schedule to be child and family friendly.

- Check that carers can manage medicine preparation and administration – ask for a demonstration.
- Serve the child's best interests – an unlicensed or off-label product may be the more appropriate choice.
- Review management regularly and recalculate doses.
- Review side-effects – they could be undetected medication errors.
- Communicate management details clearly and comprehensively – especially in 'shared care'.

References

Choonara I (1999). How to harm children in hospital – a guide for junior doctors. *Paediatric and Perinatal Drug Therapy*, 34–35.

Costello I (2007) Paediatric pharmacokinetics and pharmacodynamics. In: Costello I, Long P, Wong I, Tuleu and Yeung V (eds) *Paediatric Drug Handling*. London: Pharmaceutical Press, pp. 1–11.

Frank Shann Collective (2008) DrugDoses, 14th edn. Available at: www.drugdoses.net

FDA (US Food and Drug Administration) (1995) FDA Final Ruling 60FR13590 13 March 1995 Over-the-counter drug products intended for oral ingestion that contain alcohol. *Federal Register* 60(48):13590. Available at:
www.fda.gov/downloads/Drugs/DevelopmentApprovalProcess/
DevelopmentResources/over-the-CounterOTCDrugs/StatusofOTCRulemakings/
UCM155029.pdf [Accessed July 2010].

Gray N (2008). Helping young people to take control of their health and medicines. Presentation at the British Pharmaceutical Conference and Exhibition, Manchester Central, 7–9 September 2008. Cited in the *Pharmaceutical Journal* 281: B35.

Grießmann K, Breitkreutz J, Schubert-Zsilavecz M, Abdel-Tawab M (2007). Dosing accuracy of measuring devices provided with antibiotic suspensions. *Paediatric and Perinatal Drug Therapy* 8: 61–70.

Hummelinck A, Pollock K (2007). The relationship between healthcare professionals and the parents of chronically ill children: negotiating the boundaries between dependence and expertise. *International Journal of Pharmacy Practice* 15: 3–9.

Joint Formulary Committee (2010) *BNF: British National Formulary 60*. London: British Medical Association and Royal Pharmaceutical Society of Great Britain, October.

Kearns GL, Abdel-Rahman SM, Alander SW *et al.* (2003). Developmental pharmacology – drug disposition, action and therapy in infants and children. *New England Journal of Medicine* 349: 1157.

National Prescribing Centre (2000) Prescribing for children. *MeReC Bulletin* 11 (2). Available at:
www.npc.co.uk/ebt/merec/other_non_clinical/resources/merec_bulletin_v0111_n02.pdf [Accessed 24 March 2010].

Northern Neonatal Network (ed.) (2007) *Neonatal Formulary: Drug Use in Pregnancy and the First Year of Life*, 5th edn. Oxford: Blackwell.

Guy's, St.Thomas' and Lewisham Hospitals (2010) *Paediatric Formulary*, 8th edn. London: Guy's, St. Thomas' and Lewisham Hospitals.

Paediatric Formulary Committee (2010) *BNF for Children*. Available at:
http://bnfc.org [Accessed June 2010].

Patient UK (2010) Prescribing in children. Available at:
www.patient.co.uk/doctor/Prescribing-in-Children.htm [Accessed 24 March 2010].

Taketomo CK, Hodding JH, Kraus DM (eds) (2009) *Pediatric Dosage Handbook*, 16th edn. Hudson, OH: Lexi-Comp APhA.

Tomlin S, Cockerill H, Costello I, *et al.* (2009) Working Party. Making medicines safer for children – guidance for the use of unlicensed medicines in paediatric patients. Guidelines Vol. 37. Available at:
www.rosemontpharma.com/images/educationPDF/Paediatric%20Summary%20guideline.pdf [Accessed 24 March 2010].

Verras P, Greaves R (2005). Abnormal laboratory results: interpreting paediatric biochemistry results. *Australian Prescriber* 28: 126–129.

White R and Bradnam V (2007) *Handbook of Drug Administration via Enteral Feeding Tubes.* London: Pharmaceutical Press.

Further reading/websites of interest

World Health Organization, Royal College of Paediatrics and Child Health and the Department of Health Growth chart. www.rcpch.ac.uk/research/UK-WHO-Growth-Charts

Mind map

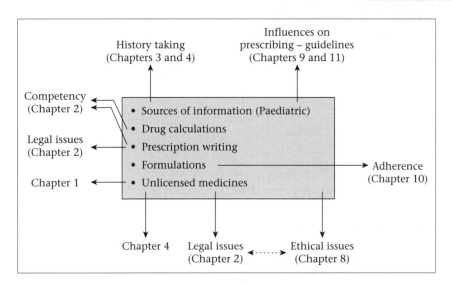

7

Monitoring prescribing

Stuart Gill-Banham

Learning outcomes

After completing this chapter you will be able to:

- understand how symptom rating scales can be used in everyday clinical practice;
- recognise potential causes and risks of adverse drug reactions and know when an ADR needs to be reported to the MHRA (Medicines and Healthcare products Regulatory Agency);
- be aware of the general principles underlying monitoring of plasma drug levels used commonly in mental health.

Introduction

Prescribing for patients with a mental illness poses some specific challenges. Psychiatry involves the detection and treatment of symptoms that are part of everyday experience; thus the prescriber may have difficulty determining whether a treatment is successful or not. However, the assessment of subjective experience is not unique to psychiatric medicine and prescribers in other fields may face a situation where monitoring the effectiveness of an intervention is difficult to judge. In general medicine, the symptom being addressed might be objective in nature, but the impact that this symptom has upon life might be much more subjective. If prescribing is to conform to a logical evidence base, there is a need to assess subjective experiences in an objective manner.

The scenario in this chapter uses a straightforward bipolar case to illustrate how objective assessment of treatment response may be achieved. Also the need for identification of rare and difficult to explain adverse drug reactions (ADRs) is illustrated along with a logical approach to managing a switch of therapy. Finally, basic general principles of pharmacokinetic drug monitoring are discussed.

Prescriber

Steven Maynard is a pharmacist who has specialised in mental health for many years. He qualified as a prescriber last year, and has been responsible for an outpatient review clinic that is based at his local community mental health team (CMHT). Individuals with long-term serious mental illnesses (SMI), such as bipolar disorder or schizophrenia are referred to Steven for on-going management of their medication. Individuals are often referred to Steven following their discharge from inpatient psychiatric care. Steven works closely with a small group of consultant psychiatrists with whom he liaises and from whom he receives advice and support.

Patient background

Derwent Baxter is a 27-year-old male who was diagnosed with bipolar disorder 4 years ago. He has had three hospital admissions since his diagnosis. On the second occasion he was prescribed quetiapine, which appeared to have been controlling his symptoms to a degree, until he stopped taking it about five months ago, when he started to deteriorate. His third, and most recent, admission to the local psychiatric unit occurred four months ago and culminated in him staying awake for a 48-hour period and disrupting the shop below his flat. He was preoccupied with the special mission given to him, in person, by Barack Obama. His mission was to engage the world in time- and energy-saving activities that will ultimately prevent the planet from destruction.

On admission to the unit a diagnosis of mania was made, which was in part attributed to the stopping of the quetiapine.

At this time he was started on olanzapine 10 mg each night. After a few days this was increased to 15 mg and then to 20 mg, as the initial response was not optimal. The quetiapine was not restarted, as it was felt that he had previously responded better to olanzapine on his first admission, than he had to quetiapine.

One week after admission Derwent was more settled, sleeping approximately 6 hours each night. He was still preoccupied with how inefficient everything was generally and, in particular, how poorly run the NHS is. It was decided to introduce sodium valproate to his regimen and the dose of this was increased gradually over the next few weeks.

After two months on the ward, Derwent was much more settled. When directly questioned about Barack Obama he would still describe having met him and he was still particular about everything connected with his care being done properly. However, he had stopped interfering with staff activities on the ward. Prior to discharge, the dose of olanzapine was decreased slightly because Derwent had been experiencing an excessive sedative effect.

He was discharged on sodium valproate 500 mg in the morning and 1000 mg at night and olanzapine 15 mg every night.

Summary sheet with background information

Name: Derwent Baxter
DOB: 11/4/*twenty-seven years ago*
Occupation: Part-time shop worker/musician

Past medical history

Admission to hospital: Diagnosed bipolar disorder *4 years ago*
Admission to psychiatric unit *3 years ago*
Admission to psychiatric unit *4 months ago*

Medication history of recent episode

Four months ago on admission to psychiatric unit

Olanzapine 10 mg at night
Promethazine 20 mg three times a day
Lorazepam 1–2 mg three times a day for severe agitation

One week after admission

Medication changed to:

Olanzapine 20 mg at night
Promethazine 20 mg up to three times a day when required
Sodium valproate 200 mg on the morning and 400 mg at night

$\rightarrow$

Over the next few weeks

> Sodium valproate gradually increased to 500 mg in the morning and 1000 mg at night

Two months ago

Discharged on current medication:

> Sodium valproate 500 mg every morning, 1000 mg every night
> Olanzapine 15 mg every night

Disease monitoring

> BMI: 27
> Blood pressure: 157/88 mmHg
> Pulse: regular 79 bpm

Mental health

On admission a mental state examination was made and found the following:

- Appearance and behaviour: Young male dressed in bright fluorescent orange waistcoat with no shirt underneath and red corduroy trousers. He appeared agitated and eager to explain how it was 'all a big mistake'. During the interview he would frequently jump up off his seat in order to see what the room was like from a different angle.
- Speech: Fast speech with excitable tone. Eager to share all of the great ideas that he had. When he felt those in the room were not listening he would repeat himself, but at a louder volume.
- Thoughts: No formal thought disorder. Preoccupied with the special mission that he had been presented with, following a visit from Barack Obama. His mission is to engage the world in time-saving activities that will save energy and the world.
- Mood: Subjectively and objectively elated. Feels that his mission is the answer to all of the world's problems and so in turn will alleviate all of his own personal worries and concerns.
- Perception: Possibly responding to unseen stimulus at time during the interview. Delusional belief about recent visit of US President to his place of residence.

continued overleaf

- Cognition: Orientated to time, person and place.
- Insight: Does not see himself as unwell, but willing to remain in hospital in order to spend time planning his mission. 'Hospital ward is as good a place as any to start saving time – maybe I can make the NHS work more effectively – they need a good organiser like me and I won't cost anything'.

Social history

Lives in flat above convenience store that a friend owns. Single, with no close family living nearby. Unclear whether he has any close relationships.

Scenario

Today Derwent comes to see Steven in an outpatient clinic for a review two weeks after being discharged. He seems to be quite overexcited, but this relates principally to his complaint about a rash over his abdomen and arms that is red and itchy. When Steven asks Derwent how his mental health is, Derwent says things have been 'fine'. In fact he has been offered promotion at work. However, he is struggling to even be at work because of 'this itching all the time'. When asked, Derwent says the rash has come on since starting the sodium valproate. 'I need to change the pills at once', Derwent insists. Steven decides to make an assessment of Derwent's current mental health and the rash before considering a switch to another agent. If sodium valproate is thought to be causing the rash then an alternative mood stabiliser will be necessary.

As a result of his consultation with Derwent, Steven decides to switch the sodium valproate to an alternative mood stabiliser, lithium carbonate. The plan is to start with 400 mg at night for a week and then to check lithium levels and adjust the dose accordingly. Derwent has not been prescribed lithium in the past, but Steven is keen to use a mood stabiliser in addition to an antipsychotic for Derwent, as previous experiences of using antipsychotics on their own have shown that Derwent has not stayed well enough for long enough. The consequences of Derwent having another manic episode at this stage, so shortly after the last, could be considerable. Potentially he could lose his job and/or his flat and there may be an impact on his relationships.

1   How would Steven have assessed Derwent's response to his current mood
     stabiliser objectively?
2   Is Steven correct in thinking that Derwent could have developed a skin rash to
     the valproate six weeks after starting it? What type of adverse drug reaction is
     this? Should Steven report this reaction?
3   Why is monitoring of lithium so important? Is Steven right to check Derwent's
     lithium plasma level after one week? How should Steven respond to the
     results of the monitoring?
4   Should Steven stop the sodium valproate immediately? Does Steven need to
     prescribe any other mediation for Derwent to cope with this transition period?
5   What other monitoring should Steven undertake with a patient on these
     medicines?

Q1   How would Steven have assessed Derwent's response to his current mood
          stabiliser objectively?

Symptoms of mental illness are often connected to the individual's internal emotions and feelings. The subjective nature of symptoms within psychiatry is not unique to this field of medicine. It may also be encountered in other areas (e.g. pain relief). Of particular relevance to psychiatry is the fact that mental illness presents with symptoms that are familiar to all, yet in a psychiatric disorder they combine, or are of such severity that they go beyond the boundaries of normal experience. The question therefore remains, how can symptoms be separated from everyday experiences, and how can a response to therapy be assessed?

A variety of rating scales have been developed for use in psychiatry. Some are for use by healthcare staff (observer rating scales), while others are intended to be completed by the individual patient (self-rating scales). These rating scales are useful in clinical practice. However, care is needed in interpretation of scores, not least because many scales were originally intended for use in clinical trials. They were not designed, therefore, to be diagnostic instruments, rather measures of clinical outcome. However, the introduction of symptom-derived diagnostic systems (e.g. International Classification of Disease (ICD) or Diagnostic and Statistical Manual (DSM)) has led to the emergence of an association between clinical diagnosis and symptom-orientated rating scales.

Rating scales enable individual symptoms to be quantified, often using a Likert scale with scores ranging from 0 (when a symptom is not present) up to 4 (when the symptom is assessed as being severe). The scores for each item of the rating scale are added and the total score should provide an overall measure of disease severity.

Self-rating scales have been developed which enable individuals to rate items of importance to themselves. The emphasis of self-rating scales may differ from that of observer-rating scales. Rather than focus upon symptom severity, issues such as social functioning, side-effects or quality of life may be assessed. There are some obvious limitations to the use of self-rating scales, particularly where cognitive function is impaired or if there is impaired linguistic ability. There is a debate as to whether items on a self-rating scale have sufficient global meaning, such that all individuals would understand the question and answer in the same way.

Reliability, that is to what degree a rating scale can produce the same result when administered at different times in a similar clinical presentation, is one of the key aspects of accuracy with rating scales. Inter-rater reliability, where different individuals should be able to produce the same results if presented with the same case, can become more difficult to ensure, the more complex a rating scale is. Reliability should not be confused with validity. Validity is a measure of how much the result produced by a rating scale truly reflects the real situation: i.e. if an individual is severely depressed, does the corresponding depression rating score reflect that?

The use of symptom-rating scales should not obscure the presented clinical situation. It would be foolish to base treatment decisions purely upon the rating score, while ignoring the presenting symptoms. The key issue is to treat the patient and not the score. With some presentations, it may be possible to achieve this and still maintain an objective approach. If an individual presents with symptoms that are a clear indicator of illness severity in their case, then the response of these symptoms to treatment can be used as a marker for response. Sometimes these key symptoms may be those that cause particular disability or impairment of social functioning. In other cases, the key symptoms may be a sign of more severe illness presentation. In monitoring response to treatment, it is important to assess the individual as a whole and not focus treatment decisions on a narrow aspect of the presentation.

In this case, the key symptoms on admission were Derwent's preoccupation with a special plan and how he was interfering with activity of staff on the ward. After admission he quickly settled, which was demonstrated by him regaining an acceptable sleep pattern. However, he remained difficult to manage and a problem for staff. The addition of sodium valproate to his medication might have been in response to this need for additional symptom control. The response to this was seen when Derwent interfered less with staff. Before discharge, the olanzapine dose was reduced slightly. This might have been in response to side-effects, particularly sedation, which initially would have been welcome but as Derwent settled more, would have become an inconvenience.

Steven could have used a brief screening tool to assess Derwent's symptoms at the time of the consultation. The mood disorder question-naire is a 15-item tool that has been shown to have good sensitivity and specificity for the symptoms of bipolar disorder (Hirschfeld *et al.*, 2000). A score of 7 or more on the scale indicates probable presence of manic symptoms.

One final important aspect of Steven's assessment of Derwent is to monitor compliance with medication. Lack of compliance is a major cause of relapse in mental illness, including bipolar disorder. The reasons why individuals take (or don't take) psychiatric medication are complex and multifaceted. A study by Gray *et al.* (2005) in individuals with schizophre-nia who were taking antipsychotics found that the majority of inpatients in one South London mental health trust were only taking antipsychotics because they had been told to by a healthcare professional. Despite this, a larger majority of patients surveyed said that they found medication to be beneficial. A study in Denmark (Kessing *et al.*, 2006) among patients with bipolar disorder found that patients on the whole did not see manic symp-toms as being part of a medical illness, rather they saw them linked to personality issues. Despite this, a majority of patients surveyed did feel that mood stabilisers make them feel stronger and so better able to deal with their problems. Compliance with medication is especially important with lithium, as frequent stop/starts can result in a worse outcome for the indi-vidual. Discontinuation of lithium, even in a controlled fashion, was found to be associated with a higher than expected rate of symptom relapse (Yazici *et al.*, 2004).

Q2   Is Steven correct in thinking that Derwent could have developed a skin rash to the valproate six weeks after starting it? What type of adverse drug reaction is this? Should Steven report this reaction?

An adverse drug reaction (ADR) is defined as 'an unwanted or harmful reaction which occurs after administration of a medicine that is known or suspected to cause the reaction' (MHRA, 2006). Such a reaction should be distinguished from an adverse event or experience. This is where an individual experiences an adverse outcome while taking a medicine, or at some time afterwards, that is not attributable to that medicine (Aronson and Ferner, 2005).

ADRs can be classified into type A and type B reactions. Those reactions that are predictable (from the primary or secondary mechanism of action of the medicine) and dose dependent are referred to as type A.

Those that cannot be predicted from the known pharmacology of the medicine and are not dose dependent are referred to as type B (Wiffen *et al.*, 2002). Examples of type A adverse reactions include: sedation (although this is not always an adverse consequence), constipation (e.g. from opioid analgesics), dry mouth (e.g. from anticholinergics, such as oxybutinin), hypotension (e.g from antipsychotics, such as haloperidol) or bradycardia (e.g from beta-blockers). Examples of type B adverse reactions might include: hepatic impairment (e.g. with carbamazepine), skin reactions (e.g. with erythromycin), neutropenia (e.g. with carbimazole) or other bizarre adverse effects such as alopecia (associated with sodium valproate).

These definitions might imply that type B reactions have no pharmacological basis, when in fact the mechanism might just not be fully understood or clear. Additional problems occur when there is overlap between type A and type B reactions. Aronson and Ferner (2005) use the example of erythromycin-induced nausea to illustrate this point. Erythromycin is known to cause nausea and vomiting in a dose-related fashion. This would make this a type A reaction. However, as this reaction is neither known, nor predictable from erythromycin's antibacterial action, then should it not be classified as a type B ADR? Perhaps classification is not as important as awareness of potential adverse effects and risk reduction strategies to minimise the effects.

Cutaneous reactions (skin-based reactions) are thought to be the most common idiosyncratic (unpredictable) drug reactions to antiepileptic drugs (Zaccara *et al.*, 2007). They can range from mild, generalised rashes (maculopapular) or itchy urticaria type reactions, to the more severe and potentially life-threatening anaphylactoid reactions such as Steven–Johnson syndrome. The rash described in this case would be consistent with it being a benign maculopapular rash, a frequent presentation of rashes associated with antiepileptic drugs (Arif *et al.*, 2007). Maculopapular rashes typically occur at the start of medicine therapy, usually in the first two months (Zaccara *et al.*, 2007). Rashes are common with some antiepileptic drugs, such as carbamazepine, phenytoin or lamotrigine, with up to 15% of patients being affected. The incidence of rash is, however, much less with sodium valproate. It was appropriate for Steven to switch the sodium valproate to an alternative mood stabiliser, as the rash was causing significant irritation, even though it was most likely to be a benign skin eruption.

Gaining information about new products is assisted by intensive monitoring of ADRs for products that have recently been licensed. When a medicine is launched, there is often only limited information regarding tolerability and safety of the product. All new medicines licensed within the UK are assigned 'black triangle' status. This black triangle is printed against the product's name in information sources such as the *British National Formulary* (BNF), *BNF for Children*, ABPI *Medicines Compendium* and in advertising material for the product. The black triangle scheme covers all new medicine products that contain a new active substance, combination of active substances, new route of administration or a significant new product indication. For a black triangle product, all ADRs should be reported to the MHRA (Medicines and Healthcare products Regulatory Agency), no matter how trivial the ADR might appear. Reports are made via the 'yellow card' reporting system. Yellow cards can be found in the back of the BNF and are also available on line (www.yellowcard.gov.uk).

After a period of time, normally at least 2 years, the safety status of the medicinal product will be reviewed by the MHRA. If the safety of the medicine has been well established, then the black triangle status will be removed. Subsequent entries of the product name in standard texts and on advertising material will then not have to be accompanied by a black triangle. For established products (non-black triangle) only serious ADRs need to be reported to the MHRA. Examples of serious ADRs include those which are fatal, life-threatening, disabling, incapacitating, or have resulted in or prolonged hospital admission, are deemed medically significant or have led to congenital abnormalities (MHRA, 2009).

Serious ADRs should be reported even if the reaction is well known and established. It is not necessary for the reporter to establish definitely that the reaction has been caused by the medicine. Suspected reactions should be reported.

Sodium valproate is not a black triangle medicine. As the rash described by Derwent fits with previous reports of rash associated with sodium valproate and is not a severe or health-threatening skin reaction there is no need to report this ADR. However, if Steven was in any doubt, then a report could be made using a yellow card. Once completed, these cards need to be sent to the MHRA. Following receipt of a yellow card, the MHRA will contact the person reporting the ADR with a more detailed report form to be completed. As a pharmacist, Steven is able to make an ADR report to the MHRA on his own accord. However, it would be advisable to contact the patient's consultant psychiatrist and his general practitioner (GP) out of courtesy and also because they may have additional relevant information to add. Steven must document a suspected ADR in the patient's record and inform the patient about the possible risks involved in encountering the medicine again.

Q3 Why is monitoring of lithium so important? Is Steven right to check Derwent's lithium plasma level after one week? How should Steven respond to the results of the monitoring?

Lithium has a narrow therapeutic index, meaning that the difference between an effective dose and a toxic dose is quite small. The difference between these two levels, effective and toxic, is sometimes referred to as a therapeutic window or index. Medicines that have an established plasma level response and a narrow therapeutic index are frequently subject to pharmacokinetic analysis. Rather than relying upon standardised dosage schemes, the dose is carefully tailored to the individual's response.

The accepted therapeutic range for lithium is a plasma level of between 0.4 and 1.0 mmol/L. Doses producing a blood level of less than 0.4 mmol/L are not thought to be of therapeutic benefit. Doses that produce a blood level that exceeds 1.0 mmol/L are likely to produce toxic effects (e.g. ataxia, confusion, coarse tremor, increasing nausea, impaired consciousness and even death). These reference ranges for lithium assume that a steady state has been achieved, where the rate of drug elimination and the rate of drug absorption are approximately equal. A further requirement of the stated therapeutic ranges for lithium is that they correspond to a plasma level taken 12 hours after the last dose was taken.

Steven is correct to take a lithium level one week after starting Derwent on lithium. He needs to wait this long to ensure that steady state has been reached. For most medicines, the time to reach steady-state kinetics is equivalent to 5 times the elimination half-life of the medicine. Lithium has an elimination half-life of approximately 24 hours. Steady-state kinetics are reached after five half-lives, that is 5 days. Often in clinical situations, it is easier to wait until one week after starting lithium before taking the first plasma level, but it could be done as soon as 5 days later.

Assuming that steady-state kinetics have been reached, and that the plasma level was taken 12 hours after the last dose of lithium, then lithium demonstrates straightforward, linear kinetics. In practice, this means that doubling the dose will double the plasma level generated in that particular patient. If the plasma level for Derwent came back as 0.25 mmol/L then the appropriate dose to aim for would be in the order of 1200 mg, as this would produce a plasma level of 0.75 mmol/L. A dose of 800 mg may be appropriate as this would give a plasma level of 0.5 mmol/L. Although this is within the therapeutic range, it is toward the lower end, and an individual who recently experienced a manic episode may require a lithium level towards the higher part of the therapeutic window.

Steven needs to ensure that the monitoring of Derwent's lithium therapy is in line with National Patient Safety Agency Guidance (NPSA) and that Derwent is given an NPSA information booklet, a lithium alert card and record book. Communication with other healthcare professionals involved in Derwent's care about the initiation of lithium is important.

Q4   Should Steven stop the sodium valproate immediately? Does Steven need to prescribe any other medication for Derwent to cope with this transition period?

Having started the lithium, Steven should not stop the valproate immediately, as it will take a few weeks for the lithium dose to stabilise. As the rash has been identified as benign, this does not pose any significant risk. If the sodium valproate was to be stopped abruptly, there is a small chance of rebound seizure activity, even though it was prescribed for a non-epileptic indication.

During the transition period, it is important to monitor Derwent's symptomology. If signs of mania start to reappear (e.g. reduced sleep, excitability, ideas regarding Barack Obama or increased desire to see that activities are organised efficiently) then a review of the medication may be needed. If the lithium is not yet at a therapeutic level, then the most appropriate action would be to increase the olanzapine back up to 20 mg. This dose had been tolerated and effective on its own, at least in holding off the more severe of Derwent's symptoms.

Once a stable lithium dose has been reached, then monthly blood tests are needed for the first four weeks. Providing that these blood results are stable, then it would then be possible to monitor Derwent's lithium level every three months.

Steven would need to prescribe an antihistamine (e.g. chlorphenamine) for Derwent while he remains on the valproate, as this would ease the itching associated with the rash. Care would be needed to ensure that the combination of chlorphenamine and olanzapine did not produce too much sedation. A non-sedating antihistamine (e.g. loratadine) could be chosen; however, the second-generation antihistamines do not tend to be as effective for itching and there may be more potential for cardiac arrhythmias. This will be a judgement call for Steven.

Q5   What other monitoring should Steven undertake with a patient on these medicines?

When prescribing medicines for the management of psychiatric disorders, it is important to consider the need for physical health monitoring. Individuals with an SMI diagnosis, such as bipolar disorder, are at increased risk of poorer physical health. Rates of metabolic syndrome and associated obesity, hypertension, abnormal lipid profile and increased waist circumference were all found to be higher in those with bipolar disorder compared to the population as a whole (Basu *et al.*, 2004). This is thought to be because of a combination of factors, including unhealthy eating habits, life stressors, effect of medication and symptoms of the illness. The National Institute for Health and Clinical Excellence (NICE) recommends that individuals with bipolar disorder should have an annual physical health review that includes: lipid levels, plasma glucose levels, blood pressure, weight, smoking status and alcohol use (NICE, 2006). In addition to general health concerns, there are specific issues linked to specific medicines that may be prescribed in the management of bipolar disorder. For individuals prescribed lithium, it is recommended that the following health checks are made before therapy is started and then at regular (usually six monthly) intervals during the course of therapy (NICE, 2006): thyroid function, renal function and full blood count. In individuals with coexisting cardiovascular disease, or those with risk factors for it, it is recommended to perform an ECG prior to starting lithium. For those prescribed sodium valproate, it is recommended that liver function is tested before starting and at regular (usually six monthly) intervals during therapy.

Scenario conclusion

One week after starting the lithium the plasma level was 0.28 mmol/L. Steven increased the dose to 800 mg each night with a further blood test requested for one week's time. The next blood level was 0.53 mmol/L. Steven decided to increase the dose further to 1000 mg each night and again recheck the blood level. This time the blood level came back as 0.69 mmol/L. Once an acceptable blood level had been reached it was possible to start reducing the sodium valproate gradually over the next couple of weeks.

Derwent's rash cleared up within a week of stopping the sodium valproate. It was a positive step for Derwent, not just because it saved him the bother of an irritating rash, but also because it gave him reassurance that Steven listened to him and acted on what he had said, 'It is really great when people take me seriously and don't just think of me as some nutter that is always making stuff up', he reported to his GP. The switch to lithium went smoothly with Derwent being stabilised on 1000 mg of lithium carbonate (Priadel) which gave a plasma level of 0.68 mmol/L (reference range 0.4–1.0 mmol/L). Some of the side-effects of lithium were a bit annoying for Derwent, particularly the increased thirst and urination. However, Steven had explained to Derwent that lithium might cause these problems and not to reduce the amount of fluids he drank if he went to the toilet more often. The polyuria occurs independently of the polydipsia and is not a consequence of increased fluid intake. Derwent was able to take on more hours at the shop, but he still remains a little way off being full time.

Prescribing pitfalls

- Don't ignore the patient. It can be difficult to decide whether an ADR is serious enough to warrant cessation of therapy, particularly if it is unclear whether that medicine has caused the ADR and if there has been a good response to therapy. Frequently patients will decide themselves what has caused a problem and even if this is out of step with the prescriber's logic it is still sensible to listen to the patient's views. After all, compliance is unlikely if the patient is adamant that their medication has caused an ADR.
- Don't be afraid to report suspected ADRs. Reporting ADRs is important as this is the only way that a clear picture of what the likely complications of drug therapy might be. Even if you are unsure as to the causative link, still report the ADR if it is a serious reaction or if the product has black triangle status.
- Don't start a therapy without first considering the desired outcomes of therapy in that particular patient. This will aid rational prescribing and make monitoring easier. If the outcomes of treatment are clear, these will fit with symptomatic monitoring or the selection of an appropriate rating scale. If the aims of treatment are not clear, then there may need to be a reassessment of the priorities, or even a reassessment of the diagnosis.
- If a plasma level is not what was expected, investigate further before reacting. Consider whether a drug interaction might be occurring, whether the patient is taking too many or too few tablets or whether the plasma level was taken at the wrong time.

Top tips

- When considering whether to discontinue a medicine because of an ADR then consider how severe or threatening to overall health it is, how much inconvenience to the individual is it causing and whether it is likely that the ADR will resolve without the medicine being discontinued.
- Type B ADRs, by their very nature, are difficult to predict, attribute a cause to, or link with any single medicine. Often it is by considering the relevant time-course of events that an offending medicine is identified. When faced with a type B ADR it is often best to find out what medicine has been most recently introduced to an individual's regimen.
- Monitoring subjective responses to medicine therapy is best achieved with a pragmatic approach. Use of objective rating scales can be useful and assist the monitoring process but they should be interpreted with a common sense, patient-focused approach. Remember whenever possible to treat the patient, not the symptom score.
- Medicines that have a narrow therapeutic window, such as lithium, will require close plasma level monitoring to ensure therapeutic response without toxicity. Plasma levels should always be interpreted according to correct pharmacokinetic principles: When was the blood sample taken? How long had elapsed since the last dose was taken? How long had it been since the dose was last altered? Has steady-state pharmacokinetics been achieved?

References

Arif H, Buchsbaum R, Weintraub D *et al.* (2007). Comparison and predictors of rash associated with 15 antiepileptic drugs. *Neurology* 68: 1701–1709.

Aronson JK, Ferner RE (2005). Clarification of terminology in drug safety. *Drug Safety* 28: 851–870.

Basu R, Brar JS, Chengappa KNR *et al.* (2004). The prevalence of the metabolic syndrome in patients with schizoaffective disorder–bipolar subtype. *Bipolar Disorders* 6: 314–318.

Gray R, Rofail D, Allen J, Newey T (2005). A survey of patient satisfaction with and subjective experiences of treatment with antipsychotic medication. *Journal of Advanced Nursing* 52: 31–37.

Hirschfeld RMA, Williams JBW, Spitzer RL *et al.* (2000). Development and validation of a screening instrument for bipolar spectrum disorder: The mood disorder questionnaire. *American Journal of Psychiatry* 157: 1873–1875.

Kessing LV, Hansen HV, Bech P (2006). Attitudes and beliefs among patients treated with mood stabilizers. *Clinical Practice and Epidemiology in Mental Health* 2: 8.

MHRA (Medicines and Healthcare products Regulatory Agency) (2006) Healthcare professional reporting of suspected adverse drug reactions. Available at: www.mhra.gov.uk [Accessed 17 December 2009].

MHRA (2009) What to report. Medicines and Healthcare products Regulatory Agency. Available at: www.mhra.gov.uk [Accessed 18 December 2009].

NICE (National Institute for Health and Clinical Excellence) (2006) Bipolar disorder: The management of bipolar disorder in adults, children and adolescents, in primary and secondary care (CG038). Available at: www.nice.org.uk/nicemedia/pdf/ CG38fullguideline.pdf [Accessed 21 March 2010].

Wiffen P, Gill M, Edwards J and Moore A (2002). Adverse drug reactions in hospital patients: A systematic review of the prospective and retrospective studies. Available at: www.ebandolier.com [Accessed 17 December 2009].

Yazici O, Kora K, Polat A, Saylan M (2004). Controlled lithium discontinuation in bipolar patients with good response to long term lithium prophylaxis. *Journal of Affective Disorders* 80: 269–271.

Zaccara G, Franciotta D, Perucca E (2007). Idiosyncratic adverse reactions to antiepileptic drugs. *Epilepsia* 48: 1223–1244.

Further reading/websites of interest

NPSA (National Patient Safety Agency) (2009) Safer lithium therapy. www.nrls.npsa.nhs. uk/resources/?entryid45=65426 [Accessed 31 March 2010].

Taylor D, Paton C and Kapur S (2009) *Maudsley Prescribing Guidelines*, 10th edn. London: Informa Healthcare.

Mind map

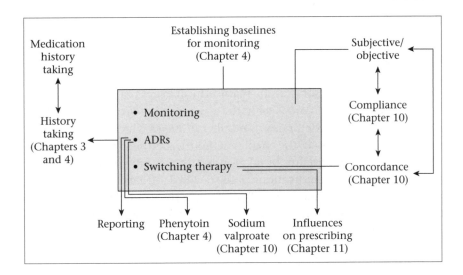

Ethical decision making in prescribing

Deborah Jenner

Learning outcomes

After completing this chapter you will be able to:

- recognise the ethical and legal aspects of consent and confidentiality in relation to prescribing;
- gain an awareness of the potential pressures that can be exerted on the prescriber by both patients and colleagues;
- respond to the needs of the patient as an individual while working in their best interests – weighing up the risks and benefits of proposed treatments.

Introduction

This chapter explores some of the many ethical issues that arise in relation to prescribing. The scenario is set in the area of palliative care, and the end-of-life situation discussed raises a number of issues which occur in other settings too. In particular, the chapter demonstrates the important issues of consent and confidentiality in relation to the prescribing of medications beyond their licensed indications. This so-called 'off-label' prescribing is a relatively common practice in palliative care. The example used describes a surgical patient who presents a significant symptom control challenge to a hospital palliative care clinical nurse specialist who is also a non-medical prescriber. It is imperative to control symptoms and to achieve the patient's desire to return home.

    Ethical issues around prescribing arise when the clinical nurse specialist has to negotiate with the surgical team responsible for the patient, advising on the use of a treatment that is both off-label and without a significant evidence base for its use. The non-medical prescriber must be sensitive to the issues of confidentiality with both carers and professionals when advising and planning care. The prescriber also has to deal with pressures exerted by the general practitioner (GP), who expresses doubts about the efficacy and cost of the prescribed treatment for which he will be responsible when the patient has been discharged.

Prescriber

Diana Harvey is an experienced clinical nurse specialist in palliative care. She worked in a similar role in the community for 3 years before joining the hospital team. A significant part of Diana's role includes advising doctors on the prescribing of medications. On many occasions, patients have a delay in receiving a recommended medicine because of time taken for doctors to prescribe because of their work commitments. On other occasions, medications would be inappropriately prescribed for symptom control needs. Diana felt that undertaking the prescribing course would enhance the care she was able to give her patients as a specialist nurse, and expedite the timeliness of treatment. She qualified as an non-medical prescriber a year ago and finds this aspect of her job both challenging and fulfilling.

Patient background

Mrs Lily Benson is a 78-year-old woman who was admitted to hospital with a two-month history of a faeculent discharge via her vagina, which was causing her considerable distress and perineal excoriation. She has a long history of cancer and surgical procedures. During the last two months she has had investigations including a CT scan and an MRI scan, neither of which revealed any obvious abnormalities. The decision was made to perform a laparotomy which revealed an obstructed loop of small bowel, extensive mucinous carcinoma and adhesions. The bowel was resected and adhesions divided, a perforation in the ileal conduit closed.

Mrs Benson was discussed at a subsequent colorectal multidisciplinary meeting and the decision was made to refer to the palliative care team for symptom control and support as she had extensive moderately differentiated mucinous carcinoma and was unlikely to be fit enough for further oncological treatment. Mrs Benson is married and has a good relationship with her husband. They have two adult children, but neither lives locally. They manage independently at home, supported by friends and neighbours and enjoy a social life, attending a senior citizens' club once a week.

Summary sheet with background information

Name: Lily Benson
DOB: 02/05/*seventy-eight years ago*
Occupation: Retired school dinner lady

Past medical history

Abdominal hysterectomy + intracavity radiotherapy *22 years ago*
Mucinous adenocarcinoma of appendix with repair of vaginal
    fistula *6 years ago*
Tumour in left colon involving bladder – total cystectomy and
    ileal conduit formation *4 years ago*
Pernicious anaemia (has hydroxocobalamin 1 mg
    intramuscularly three monthly)

Current medication

Cefuroxime 750 mg three times daily IV
Metronidazole 500 mg three times daily IV
Folic acid 5 mg daily orally when able to take (for pernicious
    anaemia)
Pantoprazole 40 mg daily IV (for gastro-oesophageal reflux)
Paracetamol 1 g four times daily IV
Metoclopramide 10 mg four times daily IV
Morphine sulphate 5 mg IV/SC 1–4 hourly as required (PRN) or:
Oramorph (morphine sulphate) 10 mg orally 1–4 hourly PRN
    when able to take
Docusate sodium 200 mg twice daily orally when able to take

Social history

Married with two adult children – both married but neither live
    locally
Non-smoker
No alcohol
Independent
Enjoys gentle social activities

Following referral to the hospital palliative care team, Diana is asked to see Mrs Benson. Diana introduces herself to Mrs Benson, explaining her role and why she has been asked to be involved. The patient was expecting a visit and is quite happy to have been referred. Diana scrutinises the medical notes, taking account of the medication history, and conducts a comprehensive assessment with the patient. One week after surgery, the patient is still feeling nauseated and vomiting a couple of times a day, despite having regular IV metoclopramide. Pain is controlled with regular IV paracetamol and topped-up with morphine as required. Her recent blood tests included analysis of renal and liver function, electrolyes and calcium levels: all are found to be within normal limits for age and the stoma is active. As a result, Diana proposes to switch the antiemetic to cyclizine 50 mg by slow IV injection three times daily as the patient is cannulated and having other medication via this route. Giving cyclizine slowly by this route should ensure the injection is not painful. Cyclizine can be given subcutaneously if necessary. There is no clear reason for the on-going vomiting, although it could be caused by the antibiotics which are due to complete in 2 days.

Cyclizine is a useful alternative antiemetic to try if metoclopramide is not effective and is often used first-line unless there is an obvious reason to indicate the suitability of another agent.

Mrs Benson is very worried; her vaginal drain has been removed and she still has a discharge. She has been advised that this should settle down in a few days.

When seen 3 days later (after the weekend), Mrs Benson is feeling better: the nausea is controlled and she is tolerating oral medication. However, when trying to mobilise, the discharge becomes much worse and is still faecal in nature. She is seen by the tissue viability clinical nurse specialist and recommendations for skin care are made. Mrs Benson is keen to go home, but feels that she and her husband won't be able to cope with the faecal discharge. The surgical team decide that they cannot offer any more treatment and the option of having carers at home is discussed and a hospice admission is considered for symptom control. Both these options are declined – the patient wants to go home.

Diana discusses the problem of the vaginal discharge with the surgical team, who are uncertain how to control it. She suggests trying octreotide, which is an analogue of the hormone somatostatin and licensed for relief of symptoms associated with neuroendocrine tumours, acromegaly and prevention of complications following pancreatic surgery (Joint Formulary

Committee, 2010). In palliative care, octreotide is often used in bowel obstruction to help decrease gastric and intestinal secretions and so reduce vomiting. The surgeons are reluctant initially as they are unfamiliar with the medicine, but Diana presents them with information from the *Palliative Care Formulary* (PCF) (Twycross and Wilcock, 2007) and it is agreed that it should be tried. They will discuss it with the patient during the ward round.

The medicine is commenced by bolus subcutaneous injection (SC) initially to gauge its effect, then given by continuous SC infusion (CSCI) to cause less discomfort and better symptom management. When Diana next visits Mrs Benson, she sees from the medical notes that the surgeons have documented that they have discussed the treatment with the Bensons, who were happy to proceed. Due to pressure of work, Diana makes a fleeting visit to Mrs Benson, who is feeling much better and looking forward to going home in the next few days. Since all seems well, Diana doesn't sit down with Mrs Benson to check on her understanding of her treatment, but does promise to contact her GP to inform him of Mrs Benson's condition and current treatment, as he will be responsible for her care and prescribing of her medication when she is at home.

When Diana phones Mrs Benson's GP, Dr Jackson, he expresses concern at the patient's deteriorating condition and acknowledges the increased medical and nursing input she is likely to require at home as her illness progresses. He states that he might visit Mrs Benson in hospital before discharge. Dr Jackson also raises the issue of the cost of continuing the octreotide, pointing out to Diana that it is an expensive medicine. He becomes quite cross, stating that he doesn't see why he should be expected to prescribe it 'on the whim of a nurse who thinks she can prescribe' when a cheaper alternative such as hyoscine butylbromide (Buscopan) could be used. Dr Jackson slams the phone down, giving Diana no time to reply. He does call into the hospital the next day and unfortunately doesn't ask to see Diana but gets cross with one of the junior doctors on the surgical team who doesn't have enough knowledge of octreotide to defend the decision to use it. The GP questions the Bensons and finds that they don't really understand anything about the medicine either, other than that it seems to be helping. He mentions the Mental Capacity Act and whether Mrs Benson is really capable of giving consent when she doesn't know anything about the treatment and the couple become upset. They are left wondering whether Mrs Benson is being experimented upon, as the GP isn't confident about the medicine's use either.

1   Diana is being required to prescribe off-label. What does this term mean? How can Diana be sure that Mr and Mrs Benson have a good understanding of the concept of taking a medicine prescribed off-label and that she is capable of giving consent? What are the implications for Diana of prescribing off-label?

2   How does the Mental Capacity Act impact on Mrs Benson's situation?

3   How might Diana best deal with the pressure being exerted on her by Dr Jackson? How might she prevent this situation arising again? Should Diana share information about Mrs Benson's care with anyone else?

Q1   Diana is being required to prescribe off-label. What does this term mean? How can Diana be sure that Mr and Mrs Benson have a good understanding of the concept of taking a medicine prescribed off-label and that she is capable of giving consent? What are the implications for Diana of prescribing off-label?

'Off-label' prescribing refers to the process whereby a medicine with a marketing authorisation (formally referred to as a product licence) in the UK, is prescribed outside of its 'licensed' indications. This includes prescribing for a condition not covered by the marketing authorisation, as in this case, or prescribing it in a higher dose, by a different route or for a group of patients not covered by the authorisation. It is sometimes called prescribing off-licence, but this can be confused with prescribing a product without a marketing authorisation in the UK (i.e. an unlicensed medicine).

Obtaining informed consent prior to commencing any medical treatment is a legal and ethical obligation and is also fundamental to ensuring patient-centred care. The main aim of informed consent is to ensure that information is provided about the potential risks, benefits and anticipated outcome of the proposed treatment in a clear and concise manner, to enable a patient to make an informed decision.

Jeffrey (2006) describes the central function of informed consent as a sharing of power and knowledge between healthcare professional and patient, a dialogue in which both parties become aware of the potential harms and benefits for the patient. The Nursing and Midwifery Council's (NMC) Code of Conduct sets out clear guidelines on obtaining consent and emphasises the need to respect patients' rights and wishes (NMC, 2008). It is also clearly stated by the Department of Health (2009) that the health professional has a duty to discuss issues with patients; the document sets out guidance on English law concerning consent to physical interventions on patients. Bridson *et al.* (2003) describe patient-centred consent to be founded on establishing the patient's objectives and sharing information rather than just disclosing it. This involves discussion and exploration of the patient's aims, fears and values, checking the level of understanding, rather than making professional assumptions.

Some patients may be reluctant to question or discuss decisions with healthcare professionals, as happened with Mr and Mrs Benson: they felt that the doctors knew best and preferred to leave the decisions on treatment to them, especially as it appeared to help them with their aim of getting Mrs Benson home.

Diana now needs to speak to Mr and Mrs Benson and explore their wishes and give as much information as possible to enable decision making. Diana must fully document the discussion in Mrs Benson's medical notes and demonstrate how, in her professional opinion, she would be acting in the patient's best interests in prescribing the medication. Diana will need to ascertain that Mrs Benson is able to give informed consent, by checking her understanding and cognitive skills through asking her to describe the proposed treatment and reasons for using it as well as the potential risks. If Mrs Benson can manage this, with some input from her husband, she will have demonstrated her decision-making capacity. Once consent has been gained, this should be documented in the patient's notes.

Prescribing off-label is both necessary and common in palliative care (Twycross and Wilcock, 2007). Indeed, up to a quarter of all palliative care prescriptions written are for off-label indications or to be given via an unlicensed route. Non-medical prescribers are permitted to prescribe off-label if this is accepted clinical practice within their speciality (Department of Health, 2006). The responsibility for this decision remains with the prescriber, who needs to ensure that the benefits outweigh the risks and informed consent is obtained, as already discussed. Parvis and Wilcock (2001) undertook a survey to inform the debate on whether it is common practice to seek consent for off-label prescribing. They found that specialists in palliative medicine did not routinely obtain informed consent, document the reason for prescribing in patients' notes or inform other healthcare professionals of off-label use. Reasons given were that the prevalence of off-label prescribing made obtaining consent impractical, discussion of off-label use could cause unnecessary anxiety for the patient or carer and some felt consent should only be sought when the off-label prescribing was not established within the speciality. The Association for Palliative Medicine and the Pain Society have produced a position statement (Twycross and Wilcock, 2007) and conclude that the Department of Health needs to assist healthcare professionals to formulate national frameworks, standards and guidelines for the use of medicines beyond licence, rather than leaving it to each clinician to determine how explicit to be. The NMC (2006), however, advises non-medical prescribers to seek verbal consent and document reasons for prescribing off-label in the patient's notes.

Q2   How does the Mental Capacity Act impact on Mrs Benson's situation?

The Mental Capacity Act 2005 provides a statutory framework to empower and protect vulnerable people who are not able to make their own decisions, particularly in terms of informed consent, patient affairs, advanced decisions and research. This framework also gives the professionals involved in a patient's care guidelines in determining that person's capacity. The Department of Health (2009) stipulates that health professionals must be aware of the legislation to ensure that people who lack capacity remain at the centre of decision making and are fully safeguarded. A patient's medical condition can have a significant impact on their ability to make decisions; if they are unwell with infection or from the effects of medication, for example, their ability to understand fully will be impaired and they will not be able to make an informed decision. The discussion may then need to take place at a later date or be discussed over several days.

The manner in which information is communicated is extremely important in informing a patient's decision. If a patient senses that the healthcare professional has time for them, is honest and open with information and imparts it in a way that is easy for the patient to understand, then a relationship of trust is fostered which is integral to credibility. The use of open-ended questions and allowing the patient to explain their understanding of proposed treatment in their own words in a supportive environment can demonstrate that the patient has capacity to make a decision. This has been described as 'chunking and checking', asking the patient to repeat the important points back to you, detailing them on paper.

It will be helpful for Diana to check that Mrs Benson still understands her treatments at subsequent meetings. Mrs Benson is an elderly woman who has endured much in the way of health problems and treatments in the last few years and although she readily agreed to the proposed treatment, she may not have understood all that was being said to her at the time. Now that the GP has started creating tension and concerns by getting so annoyed, she is unable to recall what she has been told.

If Mrs Benson had been given time by the surgeon originally and had been able to demonstrate capacity by describing in her own words the aims of the treatment and possible side-effects, including that it may be of no benefit, and that she understood these concepts and conveyed her decision to accept treatment, then capacity could have been both informed and also appropriately obtained.

Diana is able to confirm this now and will be able to discuss with Mrs Benson her desire for some control over her distressing symptoms, which would allow her to be more independent in living a normal life at home. Mrs Benson may well have realised early on that the options for gaining control of the vaginal discharge were limited, and this would have influenced her decision. At the time, she trusted the professionals involved in her care. Some of this trust may potentially have been eroded as a result of the actions of the GP. Diana will need to work closely with the family to restore this, without criticising either the surgeon or the GP. The surgeon might have argued that Mrs Benson is one of those patients who subscribes to the paternalistic view that the doctor or nurse knows best and doesn't need to be questioned. Experience suggests that many people feel this way; however, it is the duty of the healthcare professional to ensure that full and open discussions on treatment options take place with the patient regardless of their preference. It is helpful to involve the carer in these discussions, with the patient's consent, to ensure that the patient feels supported in the process.

Q3   How might Diana best deal with the pressure being exerted on her by Dr Jackson? How might she prevent this situation arising again? Should Diana share information about Mrs Benson's care with anyone else?

The prescriber must be aware of many aspects when prescribing, including accountability, consent, pharmacological issues and the influence of their prescribing on the wider multidisciplinary team. From the perspective of the acute sector non-medical prescriber in this case, this has to include the people in the patient's primary care team, such as the GP and, in Mrs Benson's case, the district nurse. When the patient is discharged from hospital, the responsibility for her care returns to her GP. This includes the prescribing and funding of her medications. In these situations the prescriber needs to communicate with the GP to make them aware of the patient's condition and the changes that have been made to the patient's care. This is especially pertinent when prescribing an expensive medicine such as octreotide, which will have an impact on the GP's budgetary constraints. Mrs Benson is not in the terminal phase of her illness, although there is no further curative treatment to be offered. It is likely that she will live for some months yet and will possibly require on-going treatment with octreotide.

Diana will need to contact Dr Jackson again and explain calmly why and how the octreotide was selected. She can run through the evidence base/lack of it with him and describe how she was hoping to trial the medication with Mrs Benson to see whether it is effective. She can invite him to ask questions, offer to send any literature she has on the use of this medicine for this condition. She should also confirm how they will work together for Mrs Benson's future best care. Diana should contact the district nurse as she will have to visit Mrs Benson on a daily basis to refill her CSCI and monitor the effect it is having on her condition. This is a considerable commitment for a busy district nurse and some notice of the increased workload is helpful for forward planning.

The issue of confidentiality must be taken into consideration when prescribing. The patient discloses personal details when an assessment is conducted on the understanding that the prescriber will keep the personal information private and not disclose it without permission, which is endorsed by the NMC's Code of Profssional Conduct (2008). However, although the duty of confidentiality is fundamental to the aspect of trust within the nurse–patient relationship, it is not absolute. There is a requirement for all prescribers to work collaboratively with colleagues to ensure effective and appropriate treatment for patients. Griffiths (2008) states that it would be impractical and possibly detrimental to the patient to obtain explicit consent each time their case was discussed, so implied consent should be obtained. Implied consent assumes that the patient understands that their information may be shared with all involved with their care. Mrs Benson was aware that Diana was working with her surgical team and consented to information about treatment being shared. In spite of this, it is good practice to keep the patient informed of discussions or disclosed information at each stage of their care. When a patient is to be discharged home, it is necessary to inform them that their GP will be contacted and advised of their hospital admission and of any changes in treatment, as the GP will assume responsibility for their care in the community. If the district nurse is to be involved, the patient must be informed of this too.

Scenario conclusion

Two days later

Diana contacts Dr Jackson and explains why octreotide was selected and states that although there is a paucity of evidence generally, there is sufficient to show its preferred use over hyoscine butylbromide. So far the medicine is proving to be effective for Mrs Benson, although Diana will continue to monitor this and feedback to the GP. The GP has calmed down, but is still a little unhappy about having to fund the use of octreotide for the foreseeable future. Diana sends references for three studies which support the use of octreotide over hyoscine butylbromide in malignant bowel obstruction and three supporting its use in controlling the output of fistulae. As those studies were conducted a few years previously, she also directs him to a more recent article (Prommer, 2008) and to the palliative care website which has a detailed formulary. Diana also asks the GP if he would like to discuss the matter further with the consultant in palliative medicine for the Trust, but he declines at that stage, finding Diana's information of sufficient use.

The district nurse is familiar with Mrs Benson and is happy to take on the extra care.

Two weeks later

Diana is asked to see Mrs Benson two weeks later in the oncology outpatient department, where she is being assessed for suitability for palliative chemotherapy. It is decided by Mrs and Mr Benson in collaboration with her oncologist that this would not be appropriate as her gradually deteriorating condition precludes her ability to cope with potential side-effects. Her main concern is that her district nurse has advised her that the octreotide CSCI is to be stopped because the supplies sent home by the hospital are running out and because it is causing site reactions and skin breakdown. Mrs Benson is understandably upset as she feels it has significantly reduced the output from the fistula, improving her quality of life and ability to cope with normal daily living. Diana contacts the local community palliative care team as Mrs Benson was referred to them on discharge from hospital. They have not yet made an initial visit, but have planned one for a few days' time.

Diana discusses the situation with the palliative care physician for the community team who advises continuing the octreotide CSCI and adding in dexamethasone 1 mg to reduce the site reaction. Diana speaks with the district nurse and informs her of the given advice. The district nurse is happy with this, as she knows the medication has been effective, but is concerned about the effect it is having on Mrs Benson's subcutaneous tissue and skin. Diana advises that the medicine should be diluted in the largest possible volume to further reduce inflammatory reactions at the CSCI site. She informs Mrs Benson of her conversations and the treatment plan and advises that the community palliative care nurse will keep a check on the situation once she has made her initial assessment visit. Mrs Benson and her husband are relieved as they couldn't face the prospect of her having to cope once again with excoriated skin and wearing large incontinence pads to manage the high-volume discharge.

Meanwhile, Diana investigates the situation further and, after consulting the *British National Formulary* (BNF) (Joint Formulary Committee,

2010) and PCF3 (Twycross and Wilcock, 2007) and discussing the problem with her consultant in palliative medicine, telephones Dr Jackson to suggest that it may be worth considering switching Mrs Benson from octreotide given by CSCI to lanreotide, which is a depot formulation of octreotide and can be given by deep intramuscular injection every two weeks. The advice from the PCF3 is that symptoms should first be controlled by octreotide. Although still expensive, the costs would be less than on-going octreotide and would improve the patient's quality of life and the district nurse's workload. The GP agrees that this is an option worth trying and will speak with the district nurse. Diana speaks with the community palliative care nurse again to advise her of the proposed treatment changes and to hand over Mrs Benson's care.

Prescribing pitfalls

- Using medicines off-label or outside their licence may be familiar to the professionals working within that speciality, but assumptions must not be made that other healthcare professionals will be willing to accept their use. Be prepared for potential opposition and be able to offer some evidence to support the benefits and risks of using them.
- When prescribing, the cost of medication is another factor to be considered. The medicines may be listed for use on the locally agreed formulary but when a patient is discharged from hospital, the responsibility for prescribing and funding lies with the GP, who may be unwilling to provide that funding. Rather than assuming the medication will be prescribed, it is good practice to communicate with the GP to state the reasons for using that particular medicine, as this approach is more likely to bring positive results.
- Prescribers should not assume that a patient is happy to continue with current medications, even if they are successful in controlling symptoms. Side-effects may be too much to cope with, so discussion needs to be on-going to deal with any concerns before they become problems.

Top tips

- Good communication skills are vital to prescribing. Discussing treatment options with the patient in such a way that they understand will enhance compliance in that medicine's usage.
- Building a trusting relationship with the patient cannot be underestimated. The patient needs to be sure that the prescriber

is working in their best interests and that it is safe to take the prescribed medication. Open and honest dialogue and showing respect for the patient's wishes are fundamental in establishing trust.

- Gaining consent from the patient to be involved in their care and ensuring they realise that prescribing is part of that involvement as a specialist nurse is vital in building a trusting relationship. Not all specialist nurses are prescribers so this needs to be clarified.
- Issues of confidentiality must be addressed and consent obtained from the patient to discuss and disclose information relating to the proposed treatment. Consent should be explicit in relation to specific treatment but can be implied when relating to disclosure. This should be checked with the patient at regular intervals or when other healthcare professionals need to be involved in the care.
- It is essential to record all prescribing decisions in the patient's medical notes, even those which have been considered but may not be used at present. It helps other healthcare professionals to remain aware of the rationale for using one medication over another.
- The prescriber must ensure their knowledge of their own speciality is up-to-date and thorough to enable appropriate use of medication for symptom control and in order to support the learning of colleagues from other specialities.
- It is useful to have knowledge of wider team working as this can help to avoid problems. Diana was fortunate to have worked in the community previously so she was aware of the pressures that other professionals have to cope with. It is helpful to know what and who is available to give care in other settings.
- The prescriber must ensure that they remain well-informed and have up-to-date awareness of current law and impending changes within the law to maintain safe practice.

References

Bridson J, Hammond C, Leach A and Chester MR (2003) Making consent patient centred. *British Medical Journal* 327: 1159–1161.

Department of Health (2006) Improving patients' access to medicines: A guide to implementing nurse and pharmacist independent within NHS in England. Gateway reference: 6429. Available at: www.dh.gov.uk/en/Publicationsandstatistics/Publications/PublicationsPolicyAndGuidance/DH_4133743 [Accessed 24 July 2009].

Department of Health (2009) Reference guide to consent for examination and treatment, 2nd edn. Available at: www.dh.gov.uk/prod_consum_dh/groups/dh_digitalassets/documents/digitalasset/dh_103653.pdf [Accessed 18 December 2009].

Griffiths R (2008). Patient confidentiality: rights and duties of nurse prescribers. *Nurse Prescribing* 6: 116–120.

Jeffrey D (2006) *Patient-centred Ethics and Communication at the End of Life*. Abingdon: Radcliffe Publishing, pp. 74–84.

Joint Formulary Committee (2010) *BNF: British National Formulary 60.* London: British Medical Association and Royal Pharmaceutical Society of Great Britain, October.

NMC (Nursing and Midwifery Council) (2006) Standards of proficiency for nurse and midwife prescribers. Available at: www.mnc-uk.org/aFrameDisplay.aspx?DocumentID=1219 [Accessed 7 August 2009].

NMC (2008) Code of Professional Conduct. Available at: www.nmc-uk.org/aDisplay Document.aspx?documentID=5982 [Accessed 25 June 2009].

Parvis H, Wilcock A (2001) Prescribing of drugs for use outside their licence in palliative care: survey of specialists in the United Kingdom. *British Medical Journal* 323: 484–485.

Prommer E (2008). Established and potential therapeutic applications of octreotide in palliative care. *Support Cancer Care* 16: 1117–1123.

Twycross R and Wilcock A (2007) *Palliative Care Formulary. PCF3,* 3rd edn. Abingdon: Palliative Drugs, pp. 375–378, xvii–xxi.

Further reading/websites of interest

Palliative Drugs. www.palliativedrugs.com. The site provides essential independent information for health professionals worldwide about medicines used in palliative and hospice care. The content is based on the UK Palliative Care Formulary (Twycross and Wilcock, 2007) which was highly commended in the British Medical Association 2008 book competition. It includes details about unlicensed (unlabelled) indications and routes, and the administration of multiple medicines by continuous subcutaneous infusion.

The Mental Capacity Act 2005. www.opsi.gov.uk/acts/acts2005/ukpga_20050009_en_1 [Accessed 25 June 2009].

Mind map

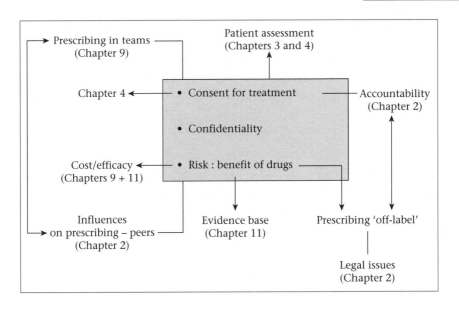

9

Prescribing as part of a team

Debbie Smart and Trudy Thomas

Learning outcomes

After completing this chapter you will be able to:

- recognise ways in which communication can breakdown within a team, compromising patient care;
- suggest ways to strengthen communication associated with prescribing in teams;
- identify potential issues associated with target-driven prescribing and see the importance of the individualisation of patient care.

Introduction

This chapter demonstrates key issues involved in prescribing as part of a team. It shows how communication between members of the team is vital and how the team can work together to ensure that the patient gets the best possible care. It also highlights the importance of individualising care for patients.

Prescriber

Richard Butcher is an experienced pharmacist who specialises in diabetes. He completed his independent prescribing programme 3 years ago. He divides his time between the local community pharmacy in the village and working as a practice pharmacist. He has just joined his local general practitioner (GP) practice on a part-time basis in order to help the practice manage its ever increasing diabetic workload. The principal GP at the practice is Dr Simon Fermat who has recently taken over as practice lead after the retirement of the previous practice principal. The practice employs one other GP and two practice nurses (one who specialises in and prescribes for people with asthma). Dr Fermat had recognised that the practice lacked expertise in diabetes. This was made especially clear to him after the recent visit from the head of medicine management at the local Primary Care Trust (PCT). The key message to Simon was, 'achieve your Quality and Outcome Framework (QOF) targets for the practice in the main therapeutic areas quickly or start looking for another job!'

When Simon first took over as lead, he did not really know what a QOF target was. However he soon discovered that this voluntary annual reward and incentive programme for all GP surgeries in England means financial reward for those surgeries who can prove they adopt good practice not only in terms of clinical care and additional services, but also in terms of organisation and ensuring a good patient experience. Good QOF results will assure the surgery's future (and Simon's reputation). Simon has put a great deal of effort into communicating the PCT message to the rest of the team. He sees it as his job as principal to make sure everyone knows how important these targets are. The previous principal did not seem too worried about such things ('his pension was safe after all'). Dr Fermat sees Richard as a great asset to (and potentially the lifesaver of) the practice team and someone who will help achieve these vital targets around diabetes, which is the 'BIG one'. Richard's focus for the next six months is to carry out medication reviews for people with diabetes and hit those targets.

Patient background

Mrs Sunita Muktar became a patient of the Rayner Road Practice in October of this year, following the death of her husband and her move to the area to live with her daughter-in-law and son. She has been a diabetic for a number of years; however, the GP-to-GP electronic record which arrived with her suggests that until now there has been a fairly relaxed approach to the management of her blood pressure, other cardiovascular risk factors and diabetic monitoring. In truth, she is not 'a great one for taking tablets'. She came to the practice expecting to be treated with the same respect she received at her previous practice, where the lead GP was a relative of her husband's. The old GP diagnosed her as diabetic and then allowed her to pretty much dictate what medicines she wanted to take after that. She saw Dr Fermat in November (last month). In her opinion he is a rude and disrespectful man. He told her in no uncertain terms that she was obese and needed to lose weight urgently and gave her pills. He said her diabetes control was 'poor' and made changes to her diabetes medicine. He said that she had to take blood pressure tablets and more medicine for cholesterol and something else . . . loads of stuff in fact. She also has to see a dietician, a foot person and a pharmacist. He even said she needed to go for walks – at her age! He then started talking about insulin injections. Sunita now has a lot of medicines and isn't quite sure which ones are which. She doesn't mind taking medicines for diabetes, that makes sense, but blood pressure is a stress thing; her last GP told her that when he popped round one evening and took her blood pressure at home. In her own environment, where she was relaxed, it was practically normal. She has been under a lot of stress recently, with the loss of her husband and the move to live with her daughter-in-law and the young children. Her blood pressure is bound to be up. It will go down again of its own accord when she is settled. Sunita hopes that the pharmacist will tell her which medicine is which and then she can decide which ones she is taking and which ones she is not.

Summary sheet with background information

Name: Sunita Muktar
DOB: 02/12/*seventy-five years ago*
Occupation: Retired

Past medical history

Reflux disease *4 years ago*
Type 2 diabetes *3 years ago*
Hypertension *one month ago*

Medication on admission to practice (GP-to-GP electronic transfer)

Nexium (esomeprazole) 40 mg one daily
Glucophage (metformin) 850 mg tablets one twice a day
Simvastatin 20 mg tablets one at night (first prescribed 1 year ago)

Repeat medication authorised by Dr Fermat

Metformin 850 mg one three times a day
Simvastatin 40 mg one at night
Ramipril 5 mg tablets one daily

$\longrightarrow$

Orlistat 120 mg capsules one three times a day
Aspirin 75 mg one daily

Disease monitoring

Height: 5 ft 5 in (165 cm)
BMI: 34
HbA1C:

| Two weeks ago | 7.9% (IFCC: 63 mmol/mol) |
| Seven months ago | 8.0% (IFCC: 64 mmol/mol) |

Cholesterol:

	1 year ago	2 weeks ago
TC	4.1 mmol/L	4.2 mmol/L
LDL	2.1 mmol/L	2.1 mmol/L
HDL	1 mmol/L	0.9 mmol/L

Blood pressure:

Six months ago	145/85 mmHg
One month ago	150/90 mmHg
Last week	155/95 mmHg
Today	150/90 mmHg

U&Es (two weeks ago): Nothing abnormal detected
eGFR: 70 mL/min/1.73 m^2 (mild renal impairment)

Social history

Lives with daughter-in-law and son
Husband died *8 months ago*
Takes no exercise
Non-smoker
Teetotal

Extracts from patient notes

One month ago – appointment with Simon Fermat

Saw pt in clinic for f/time, requesting rpt mds. Adherence – poor. To see RB for med rev once started

Adv rsks assoc with T2D/need for tight BG/BP cntrl

Inc m/formin to 850 mg tds (ac 1/12) – trgt HbA1C = 6.5 (NICE)

Strt ramipril 5 – microalb rslt (tba)

Inc statin to 40 mg to bring to target

+ asp 75 when BP u/c

Srt orlistat for wt red

Two months ago

New patient screen with practice nurse

Bloods taken – FBC, HbA1c, cholesterol

BMI 34

BP 150/90

To see Dr Fermat asap

Scenario

Richard is seeing 75-year-old Mrs Muktar today for the first time for a medication review. The lead GP, Dr Fermat has started her on blood pressure medication, and has asked Richard to see her to talk her through her medicines. 'I don't think she really understood what I was saying', Dr Fermat said to Richard. 'I suspect her compliance is dreadful. I've given her the usual diabetic, evidence-based cocktail. If you can just talk her through everything and make sure she understands the importance of taking these medicines. Stress they are literally saving her life (and ours)', he finishes dramatically.

Before Mrs Muktar arrives in the consultation, Richard prepares for the medication review by looking at her record and notes. He is finding this a little frustrating at the moment, as he does not have full access to the patient records. He has to ask one of the GPs, or if they are not around, like this afternoon, one of the reception staff to log onto the computer for him. This, and his lack of official training on the IT system, which is different from the one he has used before, means that he is unable to prescribe directly onto the system. He has to ask someone else to produce the prescription and then sign it later. However, this should be sorted by next week as the practice manager has promised to do his training on Monday (although he did say this last week!). Richard also struggles to decipher some of the finer points of Simon's notes.

A review of Mrs Muktar's repeat screen shows that Simon Fermat has started a number of new medicines for Mrs Muktar and increased her dose of metformin and simvastatin. Richard would have preferred to initiate these changes himself and go at a much slower pace. Richard strongly suspects that as it is December, Simon is thinking that he will be able to achieve QOF targets for Mrs Muktar by the PCT deadline of March. As she has been taking these new medicines for a month now, Richard can't very well turn back the clock, but he is interested to see how she is managing, given that Simon has assessed her compliance as poor.

Richard takes a careful medication history from Mrs Muktar. He goes through her repeat medication list medicine by medicine. He establishes that she hasn't started the orlistat capsules because of concerns about gelatine which she does not consume as she is a strict vegetarian. Richard is able to confirm that these capsules are made with gelatine and says he will investigate an alternative. He is relieved to find that she hasn't been started on aspirin yet, as the evidence shows that this is only appropriate once blood pressure is controlled (Ramsay *et al.*, 1999). Richard asks about over the counter (OTC) medication and establishes that Mrs Muktar doesn't take any. He is careful to reinforce Simon's messages about the importance of both good blood glucose and good blood pressure control. Mrs Muktar is convinced that stress has contributed to her recent blood pressure elevation and Richard is inclined to agree. Her BP today, however, is still raised in clinic.

Richard notes that Simon has failed to switch the Glucophage to metformin on her repeat screen. Richard confirms that Mrs Muktar still has quite a few Glucophage left, even though she is now taking three instead of two per day. He tells her that when she runs out of the Glucophage, the name of the medicine will change on her prescription. She seems a bit confused over this and Richard makes a mental note to go over this again when he next sees her in two weeks' time. Because he still hasn't got full access to the system, he is unable to alter her repeat screen himself, however he writes the following in Mrs Muktar's notes:

> *Seen by pharmacist Richard Butcher. Repeat medication discussed. No OTC meds/no allergies. Need for compliance reinforced. Using up Glucophage. Advised tds. Metformin to be added to repeat screen at next visit. Orlistat alternative needed as contains gelatine – possible diarrhoea and how to avoid it discussed.*

He also leaves a 'sticky' note on his desk which says *'Sunita Muktar NB metformin not on repeat?'* This will remind him to discuss Mrs Muktar with Simon before he next sees her.

One week later, Mrs Muktar's daughter-in-law contacts the surgery. Her mother-in-law has been unwell with a stomach bug. She is seen at the surgery by the triage nurse. The following record is made in her notes:

> *Seen by practice nurse. Unwell. Diarrhoea ++ (6 times yesterday/once today) – no N/V. Still able to eat. Prob orlistat – advised stop. Keep on Glucophage as better for GI (prob why on brand rather than generic in first place). BP 140/85. Ketones –ve, BG 14 mmol/L – checked with Molly (nurse prescriber) issued prescription for anti-diarrhoeal and Dioralyte – also issued another repeat script for Glucophage as Mrs M running low. Plan: Molly will see Mrs M with stool sample on Monday if no better.*

Monday arrives and Mrs Muktar does not attend the surgery. She is not happy that her daughter-in-law is making such as fuss. The pharmacist told her to accept diarrhoea and it is just a question of getting on with it. Everyone has told her how important the diabetic tablets are – what is a little diarrhoea to cope with? Anyway, it means she is losing weight, which everyone keeps telling her she needs to. She does not attend her next appointment with Richard either.

One month later Richard is working in the pharmacy when Mrs Muktar brings her repeat prescription in for dispensing. He works with another pharmacist who dispenses any prescriptions that Richard has written. Since Richard has not written this prescription, he is happy to be involved in the dispensing process. He immediately notices that Mrs Muktar now has repeat prescriptions for Glucophage *and* metformin. He speaks to her and establishes that she has, in fact, been taking *both* medicines for the last month. The full horror of this starts to dawn on Richard. He asks her how she has been and before she can answer, her daughter-in-law interrupts, saying 'She has been really unwell for over a month now – diarrhoea all the time, such that she hardly dare go out of the house. She is dizzy and weak and has lost so much weight. I am really worried about her.' Mrs Muktar says nothing.

1   At what stages during the scenario had there been failures in communication?
2   What might Richard do to prevent this situation from happening again?
3   How might Richard and Simon have individualised care better for Mrs Muktar?

Q1   At what stages during the scenario had there been failures in communication?

The first breakdown in communication appears to be the message from the PCT adviser, which may not have started life as 'hit the targets or else', but this is certainly how it has been received. Simon is now target-obsessed, potentially at the expense of patient care. He has also chosen to cascade this message in an alarmist way to the practice team. Simon's initial communication with Mrs Muktar was perceived by her as being rude and disrespectful. He certainly seems to have taken little time to involve her in the decision-making process. While his ultimate aim may have some basis in the evidence, his methods for achieving this demonstrate no attempt to individualise care. His notes on their consultation also leave something to be desired. While making concise notes is commendable, Simon's use of his own brand of abbreviations and shorthand have not helped the other members of the team involved in Mrs Muktar's care. Although Simon does discuss Mrs Muktar with Richard, the focus was on her lack of adherence to the 'one size fits all diabetics' list of medicines.

    Richard's own good communication is hampered by his inability to use the IT system to its full capacity. Reception staff may well have access to limited areas of the patient record and he has been logged on to the system by a receptionist. He has not understood all of Simon's notes, although he has tried to establish what is being taken by the patient. The switch from Glucophage to metformin, which would be confusing to many patients, has not been explained adequately to this elderly lady, for whom English may not be the first language and this has added to the problem. Richard's explanation of the side-effects of orlistat have also confused the picture. His notes have not made it clear that Mrs Muktar is not currently taking the orlistat. Richard has relied on the ubiquitous 'sticky' to remind himself to discuss something with Simon. This has quite possibly fallen off, or been covered by something and he has forgotten to implement his good intentions. His lack of familiarity with the IT system has meant he has not used the note-making system of the computer to ensure this message is actioned. The practice nurse has also exacerbated the situation. She has consulted the nurse prescriber (even though minor ailments and diabetes are not her speciality). While the actions may have been appropriate (because the prescription was written by someone else), there is not a full record of the prescribing decisions made.

Q2   What might Richard do to prevent this situation from happening again?

Richard needs to have full access to the patient notes. It is dangerous for him to have part access. He needs training on the system, so that he is not driving it in first gear, potentially causing problems. He needs to use the official practice messaging system to ensure that messages to himself and to others are received. He needs to be honest with Simon about his difficulties in interpreting homemade abbreviations. If he encounters official abbreviations he should ensure that he has a reference source to help with interpretation. He needs to discuss with Simon how diabetic patients will be managed within the team as a whole. Richard should ensure he also communicates with the PCT. The prescribing team are there to help all prescribers and they can provide support for the practice in achieving appropriate evidence-based interventions.

Richard will now need to report this prescribing error. There will be a local reporting system which should feed into the Reporting and Learning System at the National Patient Safety Agency (NPSA). He should discuss this reporting with Simon and the rest of the practice team. The PCT will be part of the reporting system and will want to hear how the practice as a whole will be addressing the situation to prevent future risk. Richard may also have to file a report through the pharmacy. The PCT will advise him on how best to coordinate these reports so that it doesn't look like two separate incidents.

Q3   How might Richard and Simon have individualised care better for Mrs Muktar?

A 'one size fits all' approach is not appropriate for prescribing. National Institute for Health and Clinical Excellence (NICE) guidance and similar is just that, guidance. However much the government, PCT or individuals might wish to achieve targets, patient care must be individualised within the guidance frameworks. It was inappropriate for Simon to make so many changes to Mrs Muktar's management in one go. If he was truly familiar with NICE guidance on diabetes, he would have appreciated that an HbA1C of 6.5% is not recommended for all patients and the advice is not to pursue this aggressively if it is not appropriate (NICE, 2009). Mrs Muktar is 75 years old and so far seems to have few complications of her diabetes. It may be that she will not now develop significant complications if she has had the disease for this length of time. Her greatest risk probably comes from a stroke and this is a more important focus for Richard than other aspects of her care.

Her cholesterol has not changed drastically in the last year and yet Simon has increased her simvastatin dose. Again, Simon is demonstrating good knowledge of the evidence. Studies have shown benefits with higher rather than lower doses and NICE suggests simvastatin 40 mg is appropriate for diabetic patients (unless significant side-effects occur), regardless of target. However, it appears that Simon is in an inappropriate rush to achieve the NICE target of less than 4 mmol/L. Mrs Muktar is already achieving the QOF target, which is <5 (not <4).

Simon also started Mrs Muktar on an ACE inhibitor, a decision endorsed by NICE. This is appropriate given that her eGFR and potassium levels are within acceptable limits. He does, however, put her straight onto 5 mg, when a more cautious start at 1.25 mg or 2.5 mg was indicated as per BNF. Her BP certainly seems to have dropped by the time she attends the triage nurse and her daughter-in-law reports dizziness. Although both of these effects may be related to her diarrhoea, this would need to be monitored. In addition, having been started on an ACE inhibitor, her renal function needs to be monitored.

Mrs Muktar is not uncommon in that she is demonstrating a stoic approach to what is actually a debilitating side-effect (the diarrhoea). It is possible that her inability to leave the house and the attention she is receiving from family members is part of her motivation, but there is no evidence to suggest this.

Scenario conclusion

Three months later Richard sees Mrs Muktar again at the practice. Fortunately she suffered no serious consequences as a result of the overdose of metformin. She is currently taking 850 mg metformin (as Glucophage) twice a day. Her stools have remained a little looser than before, but the frequency is only once a day and she has been happy to continue with her medication. Richard kept her on Glucophage because in his experience it can be better tolerated than the generic metformin and Mrs Muktar herself preferred taking it in the form she has been taking all along. Richard discussed sustained release metformin with the PCT prescribing adviser, who he sees regularly, but both agreed the evidence on once-daily dosing verses twice daily, in terms of compliance, was not compelling and that for the majority of patients standard dose metformin, if dose increases were introduced slowly, would be sufficient. The adviser reminded Richard that the maximum dose of sustained release metformin is 2 g and so this would not have been an option for Mrs Muktar initially anyway, although Richard points out that in practice daily doses of metformin greater than 2 g probably don't add significant benefit anyway. The switch to sustained release (SR) will be reviewed again if the diarrhoea returns, as the SR does appear to help gastrointestinal tolerability in some patients.

Today, Richard is planning to reduce Mrs Muktar's dose of Glucophage slightly to see if this will further benefit her (looser) motions. Her most recent HbA1C is 7.2% (or IFCC 55 mmol/mol under the new units). Richard is happy with this for Mrs Muktar.

The good thing to come out of 'the Mrs Muktar incident' as Richard refers to it to himself, is that she has lost 2 stone (13 kg) in weight (without resorting to orlistat). She is delighted with herself and has started to play badminton with a group of friends. The 'metformin overdose diet' is not one that Richard is planning to use with other patients, but he is happy to share his 'near miss' with other prescribers at the local non-medical prescribers' forum, for educational purposes.

Prescribing pitfalls

- Avoid abbreviations where possible in written notes. If you do use them stick to recognised ones. Read back your notes to look for potential ambiguities.
- Do not use sticky notes to pass messages on to yourself and others. They fall off and get lost.
- One size fits all prescribing is not appropriate – decisions must be individualised and reviewed regularly.
- Avoid prescribing to achieve a target at the expense of making the patient feel better. Benefit to risk ratios must always be borne in mind when prescribing and the patient involved in making these decisions where possible.
- Once-daily dosing does not offer a significant advantage in terms of compliance over standard release twice a day dosing. Modified release products may also have different licensing arrangements to standard release products. They may, however,

offer some advantages to some patients, and again one size does not fit all.

- Make sure you are fully trained in the IT system operating where you prescribe. Make sure you can operate all functions, especially those associated with passing messages.
- Ensure you have a robust system for passing messages. Never rely on your memory or the memory of others – you are relying on chance if you do.
- Record everything you do/say – if you don't record it, it didn't happen.
- Prescribing decisions must be recorded in full. This includes stopping medication.
- Involve patients in goal setting. What do they feel they can achieve?
- Ensure diabetic patients understand the progressive nature of the disease. This will help to manage change over time. Discuss insulin initiation with patients early on and put this in context.
- Try to appreciate that in the early stages of diabetes the patient may feel very well. Medication may make them feel unwell and this may have a significant adverse effect on adherence. Slow titration of doses can help reduce side-effects.
- Stepping down medication is an important prescribing decision. Stepping down may assist adherence. It may be sensible to do this at the expense of a small deterioration in other outcomes. This decision is made on an individual basis.
- Be mindful of possible pregnancy in patients with mature onset diabetes of the young. Agents such as ACE inhibitors are teratogenic.
- Some practices limit reception staff access to part of the IT system and this may be appropriate. However, they should, as a minimum, be able to put messages onto patient records. They are privy to confidential information and an awareness of the responsibilities this brings is part of their training.

References

NICE (National Institute for Health and Clinical Excellence) (2009) Type 2 diabetes. Clinical Guideline 87. Available at: www.nice.org.uk/nicemedia/pdf/ CG87QuickRefGuide.pdf [Accessed 25 March 2010].

Ramsay LE, Williams B, Johnston GD *et al.* (1999). British Hypertension Society guidelines for hypertension management 1999: summary. *British Medical Journal* 319: 630–635.

Further reading/websites of interest

Diabetes UK. www.diabetes.org.uk
Hill J and Courtney M (2008) *Prescribing in Diabetes*. Cambridge: Cambridge University Press.
Patel A (2003) *Diabetes in Focus*, 2nd edn. London: Pharmaceutical Press.

Mind map

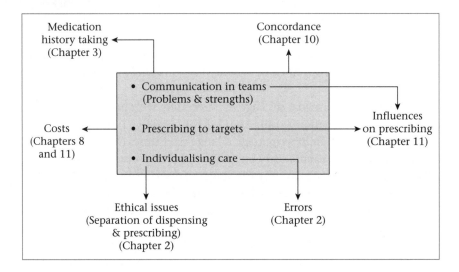

10

Establishing partnerships with patients

Greg Rogers

Learning outcomes

After completing this chapter you will be able to:

- recognise ways in which compliance and concordance affect prescribing;
- recognise ways in which the prescriber can have a positive impact on patient medication adherence;
- appreciate the importance of eliciting a patient's hidden concerns (health beliefs) about their prescribed medication.

Introduction

This scenario looks specifically at issues relating to compliance, concordance and adherence. Understanding the difference between these words helps to provide insight into the fundamentals of successful prescribing. It is estimated that up to 50% of prescribed medicines for long-term conditions are not actually taken. This represents a staggering £4.0 billion of medication left unused (Prescription Pricing Authority, 2008).

In terms of patient outcomes, research shows that 3–4% of UK hospital admissions are a result of avoidable medicine-related illness (Col *et al.*, 1990; Wasserefallen *et al.*, 2001). Between 11 and 30% of these admissions result from patients not using their medicines as recommended by the prescriber. Given that NHS expenditure on hospital admissions (excluding critical care costs) was approximately £16.4 billion in 2006–2007, the costs of admissions resulting from patients not taking medicines as recommended is estimated to be between £36 million and £196 million in 2006–2007. Adherence is a crucial subject for all prescribers. There is little point in prescribing the right medicine, in the right way, to the right patient, if they simply aren't going to be willing or able to take it. Clearly the potential cost for both patient and NHS are high if adherence isn't something that prescribers concern themselves with. The admissions figures and associated costs would be expected to decrease as medicines adherence improves.

This scenario deals with a patient with epilepsy to illustrate these points. Epilepsy has been chosen because not only is it the most common serious neurological condition but also one for which a simple omission of medication may result in loss of seizure control, with its inherent medical, psychological and social implications.

In this scenario, the patient's health beliefs are the key to the successful control of the patient's epilepsy. Compromise and joint working are needed by patient and prescriber to formulate a satisfactory medication regimen. The solution is arrived at through concordance between prescriber and patient. This is not a one-off event and adherence will need to be assessed periodically through the Quality and Outcomes Framework (QOF) review.

Prescriber

Gary Qofalot is a general practitioner (GP) with specialist interest in epilepsy. He runs weekly community clinics, to which people with epilepsy-related problems are referred. The majority have been experiencing breakthrough seizures or else problems relating to their medication. Gary is a GP by background and tends to consult in an informal style. However, when he has a full list of patients and is running behind, he has been known to rush through consultations rather too quickly, leaving patients feeling short-changed.

Patient background

Stanley (Stan) Archer is a 72-year-old pensioner, who lives alone in warden-controlled housing. His wife passed away from breast cancer 15 years earlier and he has now become used to living on his own. Physically he is fit and goes out most days for a walk to buy food and a paper. His weekly highlight is to go for a Friday night drink with his friends at the Comrades club. Since his early days of playing football at the weekends, he usually drinks around four pints of pale ale on a Friday evening. In recent years, he has favoured a local 'special brew' cask beer.

Stan developed focal onset epilepsy 4 years ago. This was heralded by a feeling of being strangely, momentarily uncertain where he was. This would sometimes lead to him smelling a peculiar odour of almonds, which on occasion was followed by his appearing blank to his friends. During particularly marked attacks, he would wander around, appearing to smack his lips in a theatrical manner. Before treatment this would be followed by a generalised seizure.

MRI scan of his head revealed some microvascular disease. Electro-encephalogram (EEG) was unremarkable. His local neurologist diagnosed him as having epilepsy, probably as a result of the microvascular disease and started him on lamotrigine. This improved his epilepsy but had to be withdrawn as it caused troublesome insomnia. Stan was then switched to carbamazepine, which has greatly reduced his seizures.

At his most recent epilepsy review, Stan's GP enquired about side-effects of medication and also seizure frequency. Stan reported that he was by and large seizure free, but every few months he would suffer from a seizure. Stan has curiously noted that these often occur on Monday mornings, something he sees as an inevitable consequence of having never liked Mondays. The GP referred Stan to Gary for some advice on this seizure variability.

Summary sheet with background information

Name: Stan Archer
DOB: 7/12/*seventy-two years ago*
Occupation: Retired laboratory technician

Past medical history

Hypertension *26 years ago*
Acne rosacea *20 years ago*
Epilepsy *4 years ago*

Current medication

Bendroflumethiazide 2.5 mg daily
Tegretol Retard (carbamazepine) 400 mg twice a day
Aspirin 75 mg daily

continued overleaf

*Disease monitoring (*from three months ago*)*

Kidney function

Sodium 136 mmol/L (136–145)
Potassium 3.9 mmol/L (3.5–5.1)
Creatinine 85 mmol/L (64–104)
eGFR (MDRD estimate): 72 mL/min/1.73 m^2

Liver function tests

Bilirubin 25 micromol/L (1–17)
AST 49 iu/L (1–50)
ALP 76 micromol/L (42–128)
GGT 109 micromol/L (10–66)

Anticonvulsant level

Carbamazepine level (random) 12.3 mmol/L (4–12 mg/L)

Social history

Lives alone
Ex smoker (35–40 cigarettes daily, but gave up 10 years ago)
Alcohol – 40–50 units a week

Scenario

On taking a full history, Gary notes that Stan drinks more than the recommended number of units of alcohol a week, most of which are consumed as part of his Friday night drinking routine. Gary suggests to Stan that these occasional seizures probably result as a consequence of drinking even more on some occasions than others. Stan stubbornly insists this is not the case and he always sticks to a maximum of four pints. He had been told when he started medication that carbamazepine and alcohol do not mix and he must be careful with his drinking.

Gary advises Stan of the risks of poor epilepsy control and suggests he reduces his drinking at least on Fridays. Gary jokes that, in spite of what Stan says, there *must* be occasions when he drinks more and this is why he is getting the seizures. When Stan starts to protest his innocence again Gary cuts across him with *'Come on my friend, I wasn't born yesterday, it's something we all do from time to time.'* Stan gets up to leave, feeling annoyed, patronised and frustrated. *'It simply isn't true'* he tries again. *'I can only help you if you tell me the truth'*, counters Gary and in a throwaway comment he also mutters *'and I bet you forget a few tablets occasionally too'*. Gary is conscious that this consultation is not going as he would like and time is pressing. He delivers his ultimatum ('patients like a straight-talking GP'): *'The choice is easy – either reduce or stop the drinking or else continue to have seizures, which would be a waste of everyone's time. I'd better get on and I will let you go away and think it over!'*

Stan is left feeling let down and humiliated after his meeting with Gary. The last thing he wants to do is to waste anyone's time. On leaving Gary's office he intentionally does not book a follow-up appointment with the receptionist. He thinks he will just have to muddle on the same as usual on his own. Stan feels a little more lonely than usual on his way home.

Reflective questions

1   What is compliance? How does it differ from adherence?
2   What clues are there that Stan is not adherent with his medication? How might Gary confirm this?
3   What do you think lies behind Stan's non-adherence? What other factors influence adherence?
4   What is concordance? Have Gary and Stan achieved concordance in this situation? If not why not?
5   How might Gary start to remedy the situation on his next consultation with Stan?

Q1   What is compliance? How does it differ from adherence?

Compliance is 'the extent to which the patient's behaviour matches the prescribers' recommendations' (NICE, 2009).

Adherence to medicines is 'the extent to which the patient's action matches the agreed recommendations' (NICE, 2009).

So what is the difference? Compliance is based on a clinician-focused viewpoint. It takes the view that the prescriber is right and knows what is best for the patient. If the patient does not do as he or she is told, this makes them 'non-compliant', which is now seen as a negative term. Having said this, non-compliance is often unintentional. Packaging that is difficult to open, misunderstanding of instructions, overcomplicated medication regimens and forgetfulness can mean that people do not take their medicines in the way that would make them most effective. This does not make the patient 'naughty or bad'. In fact, the blame for an overcomplicated medication regimen should be laid directly at the feet of the people prescribing for that patient. Non-compliance can, of course, be intentional; the patient makes the conscious decision to alter the way they take their medicines to fit in with their own lifestyle or health beliefs. We know that many people decide not to take their medicines at all.

While the terms compliance and non-compliance are now considered to be paternalistic, they are a valid measure of how medication is used by patients and because they are easier to measure than other parameters of medicine taking, they are likely still to feature in research and will still be terminology in use.

The preferred term now is adherence. This is considered to be less stigmatising for the patient. Adherence involves the patient as an active partner in setting a clinical and therapeutic course of action (i.e. incorporates the principles of concordance, which will be discussed later). Achieving adherence is important in terms of outcomes for the patient and also in financial terms to the health economy.

Q2   What clues are there that Stan is not adherent with his medication? How might Gary confirm this?

True compliance/adherence is hard to establish for definite, but asking people can be revealing. Gary did not ask Stan to say *exactly* how he takes his medicines. Follow-up questions such as 'When exactly in the morning, do you take them?' and 'Which one do you take first?' can help tell the prescriber much more about the patient and their medicine-taking habits. It can uncover all sorts of misplaced health beliefs, as in the case of the elderly woman who takes her bisphosphonate in the wardrobe every morning. Why? Because she believes she has to stand up for half an hour after taking them or she will choke to death. She has to stand in the wardrobe because she is so dizzy when she gets up in the morning as a result of her very low blood pressure, she's in danger of falling over. It emerges that she's being treated with two antihypertensives, a prescription that hasn't been changed for 5 years, since her blood pressure 'hit target'.

Asking people to bring all their medicines with them to the consultation can also be revealing: for instance, the man who wrote the days of the week on the back of his tablets himself. He did get calendar packs, but he didn't take medicines over the weekend, so he relabelled them himself, to make life easier. He didn't take them at the weekend because he got up really late and if he took his water tablets he couldn't go out for the rest of the day because he wanted to go to the toilet all the time.

Of course, some people will lie about their medicine taking and there is little that can be done about it. However, the vast majority of people will tend to tell the truth when asked a direct question about their medicines. Good rapport between patient and prescriber will make honesty more likely. The patient should be able to say 'I didn't take them because ...' without fear of incurring the displeasure of the prescriber. Likewise, the prescriber shouldn't feel upset that people have chosen not to follow the advice given. Many people will not volunteer that they do not take their medicines because they 'don't like to upset the prescriber' (because he has tried so hard or is so nice ...).

There are objective methods of monitoring compliance, such as pill counts, supervised consumption and, of course, blood levels, but these are not foolproof and unless essential, are more likely to force the patient into the 'naughty child' (who must be checked up on) role and the prescriber into the role of all-controlling parent.

The clue to poor compliance with medication in this case comes from the history of seizures. The fact that they are usually on a Monday should suggest a social cause rather than a pharmacological one. Probing Stan's views on medication would be helpful here, to gain a clearer picture. Stan has had an anticonvulsant blood level carried out and this could highlight adherence issues. However, in Stan's case, the slightly raised anticonvulsant level may be a result of not using a correctly timed pre-dose blood sample. Trough blood samples should be used (i.e. just before the next dose is due). If incorrect sampling time is suspected, a further sample should be taken before any action is carried out as a result of the level.

Q3 What do you think lies behind Stan's non-adherence? What other factors influence adherence?

There may be unintentional reasons for Stan's lack of adherence. Perhaps he doesn't really understand about the medicines he takes, how they can help someone who has seizures and how they should be taken? This may well have come out in the consultation if Gary hadn't been in such a rush. For some people, providing more information can help compliance; however, the 'chuck a leaflet at them' technique won't generally get you very far.

If a patient is suspected of intentional non-adherence, this will need to be explored carefully through a concordant consultation. The prescriber needs to gain insight into the personal beliefs that influence the patient's medicine taking. There may be difficulties relating to acceptance of the diagnosis. Patients' previous experiences and those of their family and friends will influence their own beliefs. This includes real personal experience of medicines and also experiences reported by others, the media, the internet and just perceived side-effects ('All painkillers make you drowsy'). Other influences include people's attitudes towards the professional caring for them. A bad experience with a healthcare practitioner can colour someone's view for a very long time. Stan's experience with Gary has almost certainly made a lasting impression and Gary will have to work hard to change that. Other influences on health beliefs include faith and cultural background. People's views may change over time, so that firmly held views as a young person or even at the beginning of someone's illness may be seen very differently with the passage of time.

The clue that Gary missed which holds the key to Stan's situation was when Stan said that he did not believe carbamazepine and alcohol mixed. Stan may feel that the medication is harmful in combination with the alcohol and so is choosing to stop and start his medication to fit in with his drinking. This may be because he has been previously told this is the case, or it may be that he is anticipating side-effects. However, it is equally possible that he has been suffering side-effects from his medication, such as sedation. Perhaps the combination of drowsiness from the medication and the alcohol (rather than excessive drinking alone) is causing Stan to forget his medication. Just because Stan hasn't reported any side-effects, doesn't mean he hasn't been experiencing them. Perhaps he's never been asked about them, or perhaps he hasn't been asked in such a way that has made it possible for him to answer truthfully. We know that he was offended at Gary's suggestion that he was a time-waster. Gary should have found that out about Stan for himself. Many people wish to enact the role of model patient and do not want to 'worry the doctor' or 'let the doctor down'. Eliciting health beliefs takes open questioning and time and is easy to overlook in a busy clinic.

Q4   What is concordance? Have Gary and Stan achieved concordance in this situation? If not why not?

Concordance is very different from compliance/adherence:

> Concordance is *'a recent term whose meaning has changed. It was initially applied to the consultation process in which prescriber and patient agree therapeutic decisions that incorporate their respective views, but now includes patient support in medicine taking as well as prescribing communication. Concordance reflects social values but does not address medicine-taking and may not lead to improved adherence'* (NICE, 2009).

Gary and Stan have not achieved concordance. In fact they finish slightly farther from each other's thinking than when the consultation started. In this case, it is the consultation that is non-concordant. Stan (or any other patients) would not be described as non-concordant. This is a term that is often misused.

Gary has a fixed conviction that alcohol is the only factor that matters when it comes to Stan and is no longer able to see beyond that. Also he is hurried and does not recognise that there may be other issues involved. He should have suggested that Stan come back to explore matters further when he was not so busy. Instead, in his haste, Gary has been rude to the patient, which has created another barrier between them. Gary does not convey any respect for Stan.

Stan, for his part, has not been able to express himself fully and has kept his questions and concerns internal. He also does not like being made to look ungrateful and this may prove a barrier for him to seek further medical help from Gary.

Concordance is a meeting of two experts. Gary is an expert in the management of epilepsy and Stan is an expert in himself and how he is best going deal with his condition and use medicines (or not) to help himself. There needs to be respect on both sides for the expertise of the other.

If they had been able to discuss more fully, negotiate from an informed position on both sides (Gary needs to understand where Stan is coming from) and reach a compromise, then concordance would have been more likely.

In a concordant consultation, all decisions, especially if treatment is declined, must be documented. Compromise does not mean that either party gets *exactly* what they want at the expense of the other's capitulation. Gary cannot be made to prescribe something he believes is unsafe for Stan just because Stan wants it, and likewise Stan should not have to take medicine that he is strongly against. Concordance is a dynamic process. The agreements made can be revisited at intervals and when requested by either party. Good note taking will help with this too. As in any good negotiation, a win–win situation may not be possible for both parties in terms of outcome; however, a win–win should always be achieved in terms of behaviour.

Q5 How might Gary start to remedy the situation on his next consultation with Stan?

The first step to remedy the breakdown in the therapeutic relationship between Stan and Gary is to recognise that it went wrong. People who are viewed as 'heart sink' patients may be unfairly labelled as such when the problem originally generated from a non-concordant consultation, such as this one. To make a fresh start it may perhaps help to apologise to Stan that the last appointment was hurried. Setting aside time during the appointment for Stan to say what is on his mind will also be beneficial. Open questions are helpful here and, if applicable, open invitations to challenge what was said before. For example, Gary could try 'I got the feeling last time that I had not quite got to the bottom of the problem' or 'I have a hunch you might have been holding something back'.

Asking Stan a question, such as 'How many tablets a week/month/ year would you occasionally miss out inadvertently?', will go some way in helping a patient to report truthfully. It says 'We are all human and every-one forgets at times'. Explaining clearly the diagnosis and aetiology of the illness and how medicines help to manage this should also enable patients to judge for themselves as to whether taking a particular medicine is worth-while. Written back-up information can also help people to remember what was said and give the time to consider matters outside the stressful confines of an appointment.

Scenario conclusion

Later that evening Gary reflects on his consultation with Stan. He knows he has let Stan down. It was hard to read what was on his mind; however, that shouldn't have stopped Gary from trying. Gary follows up Stan's notes the next day, still feeling uneasy. He notes that Stan's sodium level was on the low side of normal, although Gary recognises that this was likely to be the result of taking carbamazepine. The GGT was raised and in light of the history of drinking alcohol to excess, Gary naturally concluded that this was affecting Stan's liver. He now realises that incorrect timing of the carbamazepine dose has made the result meaningless. Gary decides to send a letter to Stan explaining that his recent results are slightly outside the normal range and offering him an appointment at the end of a clinic, stressing that he will be less busy.

The letter is received by Stan with mixed emotions but he feels obliged to attend. Gary starts by apologising for being rather hurried last time and explains that he was keen to reduce the number of seizures Stan is experiencing. Gary also explains that one of the blood results is an early warning sign of long-term alcohol toxicity, but as the other liver tests were normal, there was hope that this will reduce to the normal range if Stan is able to curb his alcohol intake. This advice is fully taken on board by Stan, who had wondered to himself if it would be a good idea to reduce his drinking. 'I would need some help . . .', he adds quietly. Gary is happy to support Stan.

The following year

Stan's liver tests have improved and the carbamazepine level is satisfactory in the upper end of the therapeutic range. Stan is now sticking to a maximum of two pints of pale ale on his Friday nights out. However, occasional Monday morning seizures continue. Gary is confident that medication is being taken regularly, as a recent pre-dose blood level was normal. At a loss and ignoring the clock, Gary then openly admits that something else must be happening to explain why things have not completely settled. Does Stan have any ideas himself?

Stan is happy to be included in solving the mystery. He reveals that the link between alcohol and epilepsy has always worried him, so to be on the safe side he tends not to take his carbamazepine on Fridays and only start it when he is sure he has let his drink wear off. This could be Saturday night or occasionally Sunday morning.

Gary advises Stan that this is the most important time to take the carbamazepine and rather than stop it he would come to no harm taking it then; indeed, of all the days of the week this is the time when his seizure threshold would be most challenged. Stan looks stunned. Gary gives him a leaflet on alcohol and epilepsy (from Epilepsy Action) to take home and digest at his leisure.

Six months later

The advice Gary gave Stan last time made sense and he has acted on it. He has stopped missing out his tablets when he drinks on a Friday and at last he is seizure free.

Prescribing pitfalls

- When a person with epilepsy appears to have been well controlled for a while and then has periods of lack of control don't forget to think about adherence.
- Don't change medicine doses based on the results of one test. Be suspicious about the test and get it repeated. If it is still unusual, explore adherence before reaching for the prescribing pad.
- Avoid seeing a person's refusal to take their medication as a personal affront. It is perfectly possible for a consultation between healthcare professional and patient to be concordant even if both parties disagree. There may not be a 'win–win' in terms of outcome but there can be a

'win–win' in terms of behaviour and the door is open to further discussion.

- Don't be afraid of the expert patient. With time, most patients become knowledgeable on their illness and many are up to date with current research. The expert patient programme is a valuable resource for people with long-term conditions and blogs on support group websites, such as Epilepsy Action in this case, can often be very helpful in sharing practical help. All members of the primary healthcare team can be involved with this education process.

Top tips

- The prescriber should view a consultation as the synthesis of a shared treatment design where the person with epilepsy is fully committed to the final treatment plan. If this is a compromise after a patient admits to being non-adherent and declines advice to change the practice, thereby putting them at risk, clear medico-legal notes are necessary. Ideally a copy is given to the patient whereby the discussion and conclusion can be reviewed in their own time and pace.
- Good notes also enable the conversation to be picked up and developed further at the next review. To be non-judgemental here is vital, as the door can be left open for the patient to come back and pick up the conversation rather than dread a sanctimonious consultation with their clinician.
- Allow more time, if possible, for the initial prescribing of a new medication. This will enable the patient time to ask questions and for the implications to sink in.

References

Col N, Fanale JE, Kronholm P (1990) The role of medication non-compliance and adverse drug reactions in hospitalisations of the elderly. *Archives of Internal Medicine* 150: 841–845.

NICE (National Institute for Health and Clinical Excellence) (2009) Medicines adherence. CG 76. Available at: www.nice.org.uk/CG76. [Accessed 13 December 2009].

Prescription Pricing Authority (2008) Update on growth in prescription volume and cost in the year to March 2008. Prescription Pricing Authority.

Wasserefallen JB, Livio F, Buclin T *et al.* (2001) Rate, type and cost of adverse drug reactions in emergency department admissions. *European Journal of Internal Medicine* 12: 442–447.

Further reading and websites of interest

Bub B (2005) *Communication Skills that Heal. A practical approach to a new professionalism in medicine.* Oxford: Radcliffe Publishing.

Epilepsy Action (2010). www.epilepsy.org.uk/

National Society for Epilepsy. www.epilepsysociety.org.uk/Homepage

NICE (National Institute for Health and Clinical Excellence) (2004) The epilepsies: the diagnosis and management of the epilepsies in adults and children in primary and secondary care. http://guidance.nice.org.uk/CG20 [Accessed 13 December 2009].

Mind map

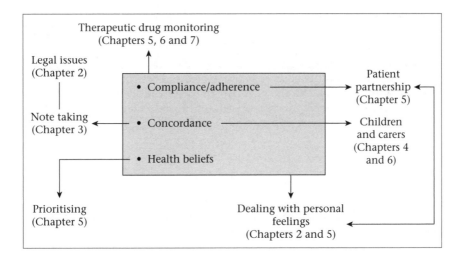

11

Influences on prescribing

Hilary Pinnock

Learning outcomes

After completing this chapter you will be able to:

- know how to apply guideline recommendations in clinical practice;
- be able to assess the balance between cost and benefit;
- know how to navigate and negotiate the diverse influences to reach an appropriate, agreed prescribing plan for the individual.

Introduction

This chapter considers the many and diverse influences that affect prescribing decisions in the context of treatment for poorly controlled asthma. Sources of evidence-based knowledge have to be identified, guideline recommendations have to be assessed for applicability, and pressures for cost containment have to be balanced against effectiveness in the individual clinical situation. In addition, the patient brings their preferences, preconceived ideas and concerns which need to be acknowledged and considered as a treatment plan is negotiated.

Prescriber

Dr Helen Brown is a general practitioner (GP) trainer who works in a purpose-built medical centre in a small market town with four full-time partners, a part-time salaried GP and three nurses, one of whom has an asthma diploma and is a prescriber. Patients are encouraged normally to see their 'own GP', so over the 25 years she has been in the practice,

Helen has been providing continuity of care to her patients and their families.

Patient background

Laura Roberts is a 53-year-old woman who, until recently, would have said that she enjoyed good health. She likes her work as a personal assistant to the manager of an expanding local business and, after 15 years with the company, is an influential and respected member of the team.

She has had asthma since childhood, but since reaching adulthood has not really been troubled by symptoms. Exercise (which she avoids) triggers wheeze, and she only used regular 'preventer' medication 'when she needed it' (which was usually only for a few weeks after a viral upper respiratory tract infection). She always carried a 'reliever' inhaler in her handbag and kept spares at work and in the car 'just in case'.

Last autumn several things seemed go wrong. A cold, which she caught from her young grand-daughter, triggered an asthma attack, and she needed a course of steroids for the first time in some years. When she tried to stop her beclometasone a few weeks later, her symptoms recurred. She booked a telephone consultation with the asthma nurse who had explained how 'preventer' treatment works and advised Laura to stay on a maintenance dose of beclometasone 200 micrograms twice a day, delivered by pressurised metered dose inhaler (pMDI) with salbutamol pMDI 2 puffs as needed. Although this helped, it did not stop all the symptoms and Laura was still using the salbutamol inhaler several times a day.

Coincidentally, three other health problems had arisen at the same time. Routine screening by her optician had detected early glaucoma and she was now using regular eye drops to control the intra-ocular pressure. She had wrenched her right shoulder doing some heavy gardening and was buying painkillers, which she took when needed. In addition, at 53 years of age, she was not surprised that she was developing menopausal symptoms. Becoming somewhat frustrated by her on-going symptoms, she decided to book an appointment with Dr Brown, her GP for the last 20 years.

Summary sheet with background information

Name: Laura Roberts
DOB: 15/7/*fifty-three years ago*
Occupation: Personal assistant to the manager of a local company

Past medical history

Asthma since childhood
Glaucoma 15 months ago
Allergies: Grass pollen

Current medication

Clenil Modulite (beclometasone dipropionate) 200 micrograms
    1 puff twice a day (last dispensed *six weeks ago*)
Salbutamol 100 micrograms CFC-free pMDI 2 puffs 4–6 hourly as
    required (last dispensed *two weeks ago*)
Dorzolamide 2% eye drops twice daily to affected eye

Past medication

Beclometasone pMDI 200 micrograms 1 puff twice a day
    (changed by the practice eight months ago to Clenil Modulite
    200 micrograms twice a day)
Ibuprofen 400 mg (OTC) one three times a day when required for
    pain

Disease monitoring

	Today	18 months ago	2 years ago
Standard morbidity questions (Pearson and Bucknall, 1999):			
Have you had difficulty sleeping because of asthma symptoms (including cough)?	Yes	No	No

$\rightarrow$

	Today	18 months ago	2 years ago
Have you had your usual asthma symptoms during the day (cough, wheeze, chest tightness or breathlessness)?	Yes	Yes	Yes
Has your asthma interfered with your usual activities (e.g. housework, work, school, etc.)?	Yes	No	No
Number of salbutamol inhalers prescribed in the last six months	8	2	3
Number of exacerbations needing oral steroids in the last year	1	0	0

Inhaler technique assessed as adequate *(2 years ago)*

Other investigations

Haemoglobin (checked two months previously with routine blood tests for the ophthalmology outpatient clinic) = 12.6 g/dL (12–15)

Social history

Married with two adult children and three grandchildren
Ex-smoker (quit with her second pregnancy 25 years ago)
Busy and active, but takes little exercise

Laura explains to Dr Brown that the most important issue for her is the asthma, but she is also hoping to mention her persistent shoulder pain and the hot flushes which have been a nuisance recently. After describing the trouble she is having with her respiratory symptoms, Laura suggests that the problem might be because her 'preventer' inhaler had been changed recently (it was now called Clenil) and although she can see that it contains the same medicine, she wonders if it is a 'cheap alternative' that is not so effective. She had discussed the problem with a friend who told her about a tablet which had helped his asthma when it had been particularly trouble-some during the hay fever season. Laura is also allergic to grass pollen and wonders if this will help her too.

Helen asks some specific questions about the asthma symptoms and elicits that Laura is having symptoms most days, that they are beginning to interfere with her normal activities and that, although she isn't sure whether it is the asthma or hot flushes that are disturbing her sleep, she often uses her salbutamol inhaler to make her chest more comfortable before she goes back to sleep. It is not clear why Laura is experiencing asthma symptoms since the exacerbation the previous autumn. She has recently been exposed to dust and fumes as a result of an extensive refur-bishment at work. Poor asthma control is often due to incorrect inhaler technique, though Helen noted that Laura's pMDI technique had been assessed as adequate two years previously.

Reflective questions

1   What guidelines are available that could help Helen decide on the best treatment for Laura? How should the recommendations be used to inform prescribing decisions?
2   Why was Laura's beclometasone inhaler recently switched to Clenil Modulite?
3   Laura has been discussing her asthma with a friend who suggested she should ask about a tablet that had helped him when his asthma flared up in the hay fever season. How should Helen respond to this question?

Q1   What guidelines are available that could help Helen decide on the best treatment for Laura? How should the recommendations be used to inform prescribing decisions?

National and international guidelines are available for most common conditions, including asthma (Global Initiative for Asthma, 2007; BTS-SIGN, 2009). Helen can access these from her surgery computer. Key sources of guidelines in the UK are the National Institute for Health and Clinical Excellence (NICE) and the Scottish Intercollegiate Guideline Network (SIGN), but if she is unsure which is the latest guideline, Helen can use a portal, such as NHS Evidence (www.nice.org.uk/nhsevidence/) to search across the range of databases and guideline collections for relevant information.

Most evidence-based guidelines are developed according to processes that adhere to internationally agreed quality standards (The AGREE

Collaboration, 2001). The methodology involves devising standardised questions, systematically searching and retrieving literature (SIGN, 2008; NICE, 2009). All relevant papers are critically appraised, normally by two reviewers, according to a protocol, data are extracted and evidence tables compiled. Multidisciplinary groups then review and judge the quality of the evidence before developing recommendations which are graded according to the strength of evidence on which they are based.

Grades of recommendations

When Helen checks the BTS-SIGN asthma guideline (2009) she will notice that there is a grade A recommendation that 'the first choice as add-on therapy to inhaled steroids is a long-acting beta$_2$-agonist' for adults uncontrolled on 400 micrograms of beclometasone a day. She will also see that the advice about other treatments (e.g. a leukotriene receptor antagonists) is ungraded. This highlights some of the more important caveats to evidence-based guidelines. Grade A evidence depends on there being a 'body of well-conducted trials and/or meta-analyses' such as exists for long-acting beta$_2$-agonists (SIGN, 2008). Lack of the evidence needed for a grade A recommendation does not mean that the medicine is ineffective; only that at the time of the guideline development, there was insufficient evidence to draw a conclusion. It is, of course, possible to have grade A evidence that an intervention does not work (e.g. air ionisers do not benefit asthma (BTS-SIGN, 2009)).

Application to the individual patient

Informed by the guideline, Helen and Laura will now have to decide if the recommendation is relevant to Laura's situation. There are several considerations which need to be taken into account.

Co-morbidity

Guidelines are disease specific, and the trials on which they are based often recruit people from a limited age range and will usually have narrow entry criteria designed to exclude people with co-morbidity. In Laura's case, the asthma guideline would appear to be appropriate. She has been a smoker, although she quit 25 years ago. This was after about 8 years of smoking 10 cigarettes a day, so significant chronic obstructive pulmonary disease would seem unlikely. Her cardiovascular system is normal and a recent haemoglobin was 12.6 g/dL, thus excluding other common causes of breathlessness.

Triggers

Laura knows that she is allergic to grass pollen and will need advice about nasal steroids in the hay fever season, but she has no symptoms of rhinitis at the moment. She was diagnosed with glaucoma at about the time her asthma deteriorated and Helen is aware that beta-blocker eye drops can exacerbate asthma. However, a check on her prescribing record shows that Laura is using dorzolamide eye drops, which are safe. Some people (about 1 in 20) with asthma are intolerant of aspirin and non-steroidal anti-inflammatory medicines, and Laura has been buying ibuprofen for her painful shoulder. Helen is reassured to hear that Laura has used ibuprofen for many years without ill effect.

Q2   Why was Laura's beclometasone inhaler recently switched to Clenil Modulite?

Some months ago, when she collected her prescription from the pharmacist, Laura discovered that her usual beclometasone pMDI had been changed to the 'CFC-free' Clenil Modulite. Although the note that had accompanied the switch reassured her that it was only the propellant that was different, she was concerned that her worsening asthma may be caused by this change.

Such switches are undertaken by practices for a number of reasons. Withdrawal of an existing preparation may force a change, or new safety information may make a change necessary. Primary Care Organisations (PCOs) often run prescribing incentive schemes which, based on evidence of good practice and health economic data, reward practices which change their prescribing in line with the scheme. In this case, it was the international ban on chlorofluorocarbons (CFCs) that had necessitated a switch to a CFC-free inhaler. With advice from the PCO pharmacy advisor, Helen's practice had implemented a process to achieve an efficient transition to cost-effective alternatives. In general, the switch had progressed uneventfully; however, for Laura, who had not attended an asthma review since then, there had not been the opportunity to discuss the change and consider the alternatives.

The practice computer system is an important tool in prompting cost-effective prescribing. Changing from branded products to the (usually cheaper) generic is part of usual prescribing packages, though it is a feature that needs to be used appropriately. In Laura's case she has been switched from generic beclometasone to branded Clenil because there is not dose equivalence across all CFC-free beclometasone products and the *British National Formulary* (BNF) advises prescribing by brand, to ensure the patient receives a consistent formulation (Joint Formulary Committee, 2010). Many PCOs are encouraging practices to use an 'add-on' programme which interrupts the prescribing process, offering cost-effective alternatives to the chosen medicine. In addition, practices can customise their system to offer an initial limited selection of medicines to encourage clinicians to prescribe in line with locally agreed formularies.

Q3   Laura has been discussing her asthma with a friend who suggested she should ask about a tablet that had helped him when his asthma flared up in the hay fever season. How should Helen respond to this question?

The most recently introduced oral treatment for asthma is montelukast, and Laura's question raises some interesting considerations for Helen. She has seen some data from a pharmaceutical company representative which looked impressive, though she is aware of the dangers of accepting marketing information uncritically.

Interpreting trial data

A crucial first step in interpreting trial data is to check whether the trial population is relevant. A trial conducted on, say, teenagers attending a tertiary care allergy centre cannot be assumed to be directly transferable to an adult primary care population. Another common pitfall is the failure to distinguish between a statistically significant difference and a clinically significant benefit. For example, a trial might show a statistically significant difference of, say, 10 L/min in morning peak flow, but this is such a small difference that it may be of little benefit clinically. In addition, trial data are usually presented as 'group mean data' (i.e. the average by which the group of participants changed). This does not imply that everyone given the treatment will benefit by the average 10 L/min. Some participants may have responded very well and gained 100 L/min, while others have deteriorated by 60 L/min. Trials increasingly use patient reported outcome measures (such as symptom or quality of life scores) which may be of more relevance to patients than measures of lung function.

Helen's previous experience with montelukast was that it seemed to benefit some people better than others. The fact that Laura's friend had hay fever may be relevant, as montelukast improves nasal symptoms as well as asthma, so both aspects of his condition may have benefitted.

The patient's perspective

Patients will often have ideas about the treatment they would like to try and these should be discussed and, if clinically appropriate, accommodated as this is likely to improve compliance. As Helen discovered when she read the asthma guidelines, there is a choice of add-on therapy for asthma and Laura's interest in the tablet her friend had used successfully can be put into the perspective of guideline recommendations.

Information from the internet and health stories (or scares) in the media are other important influences. In the context of asthma, a common problem is that the reporting of the side-effects of oral steroids (often confused with anabolic steroids taken by athletes) may concern people prescribed inhaled glucocorticoid steroids for asthma. In the UK 'direct to patient' advertising is not allowed, but pharmaceutical companies can fund media campaigns to promote awareness of a condition. Advertising montelukast would therefore not be allowed, but a campaign to raise awareness of the link between rhinitis and asthma and the availability of treatments to help both conditions would probably be acceptable and might influence Laura's request.

Patients expect their ideas to be taken seriously and normally a discussion in which their suggestions about treatment options are balanced with clinical information from guidelines and the experience of their professional adviser, will result in an agreed course of action. Occasionally, however, patients will persist in demanding a prescription for a treatment that the clinician believes is inappropriate. Medicolegally, a prescription represents the considered opinion of the prescriber that the medicine is appropriate treatment for the patient's current clinical condition: if the clinician is not satisfied that this is the case, they should refuse to prescribe. Requesting the advice of a mutually recognised expert may be a useful strategy for avoiding outright confrontation.

The scenario continues

Helen and Laura decide to follow the recommendation in the asthma guideline and to commence a trial of treatment with a long-acting beta$_2$-agonist. Having taken this decision, there are more aspects of prescribing to consider.

Reflective questions

4   What might influence Helen's choice of inhaler device for Laura?
5   What other information might impact on the advice that Helen gives Laura?

Q4   What might influence Helen's choice of inhaler device for Laura?

Helen is aware of guidance recommending pMDIs as the most cost-effective option (Brocklebank *et al.*, 2001), and that the local PCO prescribing incentive scheme was monitoring the use of the more expensive devices. She is also aware that if Laura cannot use a pMDI then the medicine would not work for her, which could prove more expensive in the long term as her asthma would remain out of control. However, after a reminder not to inhale too fast, Helen assesses Laura's pMDI inhaler technique as satisfactory and prescribes formoterol pMDI 12 micrograms twice a day.

Long-acting beta$_2$-agonists can be prescribed in a combination inhaler with an inhaled steroid which has the advantage of convenience for the patient (and a cost saving for Laura who pays prescription charges). It will also ensure one medicine cannot be taken without the other. A disadvantage of combination products is that they prevent flexible adjustment of individual medicine within the combination so that stepping treatment up or down is more difficult. As Laura's asthma is currently poor, Helen and Laura decide she should start with individual inhalers until she is sure the treatment has worked and that she is using the optimal dose, but that a combination could be considered in the future if long-term add-on treatment is needed.

Q5   What other information might impact on the advice that Helen gives Laura?

Helen remembers a warning from the Medicines and Healthcare products Regulatory Agency (MHRA) about long-acting beta$_2$-agonists, which had recently investigated concerns about an excess in fatal asthma attacks in patients taking salmeterol or formoterol (MHRA, 2005). This very small risk, which is reduced in patients using concomitant inhaled steroids, needs to be balanced against the substantial benefits of long-acting beta$_2$-agonists on symptom control and exacerbation rate. Remembering that until recently Laura has tended to take inhaled steroids intermittently, Helen emphasises the importance of continuing regular treatment with Clenil along with the new add-on therapy.

Scenario conclusion

Helen recommends that Laura attends the practice asthma clinic for follow-up. The asthma nurse is pleased to learn that her symptoms are much reduced and discusses combining her two treatments in one inhaler. Three months later, the asthma nurse reports that Laura is now controlled on a beclometasone/formoterol pMDI inhaler which she takes regularly twice a day. At that clinic visit, the nurse reviewed Laura's Asthma Action Plan and amended it to take account of the new treatment. Her plan is to see Laura again in another three months, with a view to plan her step down as per BTS-SIGN guidelines, assuming her asthma remains well controlled.

Prescribing pitfalls

- Don't be misled by 'grades of recommendation' in guidelines. The grade allocated depends on how much high-quality evidence is available, not whether a treatment is effective.
- Don't use PCO (or any other) incentive schemes blindly. They can be useful aids to cost-effective prescribing, but their recommendations will not be right for all patients under all circumstances.
- Don't forget to question pharmaceutical company advice. Pharmaceutical companies act within the regulatory framework of the Association of the British Pharmaceutical Industry, which means they should not be misleading or inaccurate. However, you should not take everything at face value and should be prepared to ask for more information. It is helpful to put pharmaceutical company advice into perspective using unbiased systematic reviews or guidelines.
- Don't forget there is a distinction between a statistically significant benefit and a clinically significant difference.
- Don't forget medicine side-effects. Always ask about other medication, including treatments bought over the counter.
- Don't assume compliance. Many (if not all) patients will adapt their use of treatment to suit their perceived needs.
- Don't commit to long-term prescribing until a trial of treatment has shown that the treatment strategy is beneficial and does not cause troublesome side-effects.

Top tips

- Do make use of available guidelines. Portals such as NHS Evidence (http://www.nice.org.uk/nhsevidence/) provide access to a range of databases and guideline collections.
- Do remember that guidelines make recommendations for the 'average patient in the average situation' – they will not be right for every patient in every situation.
- Do remember that every patient is different. Some respond well to a treatment: others do not benefit. Some will experience side-effects; others do not.
- Do remember that practice-based medicine switches might be a pragmatic necessity, but they can cause anxiety. Ensure that

there are adequate mechanisms to enable concerned patients to seek advice.

- Do remember that patients have many sources of information. Family and friends offer advice, and newspapers, magazines and the internet provide information which should be discussed in the light of the clinician's knowledge to reach a negotiated treatment plan.
- Do use available prescribing tools. The practice computer system facilitates compliance with the practice formulary, prompts cost-effective prescribing and incorporates safety checks.
- Do remember that a change of treatment may necessitate a change in self-management advice.

References

BTS-SIGN (British Thoracic Society-Scottish Intercollegiate Guideline Network) (2009) British guideline on the management of asthma. Available at: www.brit-thoracic.org.uk/clinical-information/asthma/asthma-guidelines.aspx [Accessed 27 March 2010].

Brocklebank D, Ram F, Wright J *et al.* (2001) Comparison of the effectiveness of inhaler devices in asthma and chronic obstructive airways disease: a systematic review of the literature. *Health Technology Assessment* 5: 1–149.

Global Initiative for Asthma (2009) Global strategy for asthma management and prevention. Available at: www.ginasthma.org [Accessed 13 August 2010].

Joint Formulary Committee (2010) *BNF: British National Formulary 60*. London: British Medical Association and Royal Pharmaceutical Society of Great Britain.

MHRA (Medicines and Healthcare products Regulatory Agency) (2005) Reminder: salmeterol (Serevent) and formoterol (Oxis, Foradil) in asthma management. November 2005. Available at: www.mhra.gov.uk/Safetyinformation/Safetywarningsalertsandrecalls/Safetywarningsandmessagesformedicines/CON2022601 [Accessed June 2010].

NICE (National Institute for Health and Clinical Excellence) (2009) *The Guidelines Manual*. London: NICE.

Pearson MG and Bucknall CE (eds) (1999) *Measuring Clinical Outcome in Asthma: A patient-focused approach*. London: Royal College of Physicians.

SIGN (Scottish Intercollegiate Guideline Network) (2008) *SIGN 50: A Guideline Developer's Handbook*. Edinburgh: SIGN.

The AGREE Collaboration (2001) The Appraisal of Guidelines for Research and Evaluation (AGREE) instrument. Available at: www.agreetrust.org [Accessed 1 March 2009].

Further reading/websites of interest

Web-portals

Bandolier – Evidence-Based Healthcare. www.jr2.0x.ac.uk/bandolier/index.html

Centre for Evidence-Based Child Health. www.ich.ucl.ac.uk/ich/html/academicunits/paed_epid/cebch/about.html

Centre for Evidence-Based Medicine. www.medlib.iupui.edu/ebm/home.html

Centre for Reviews and Dissemination. www.york.ac.uk/inst/crd/

National Guideline Clearinghouse (NGC), a public resource for evidence-based clinical practice guidelines. www.guideline.gov/index.aspx

NHS evidence is a web-based service that provides easy access to high-quality clinical and non-clinical information about health and social care. www.nice.org.uk/nhsevidence/

Guidelines

The National Institute of health and Clinical Excellence (NICE) is an independent organisation responsible for providing national guidance on promoting good health and preventing and treating ill health. www.nice.org.uk/

Scottish Intercollegiate Guideline Network (SIGN) (2010) develops and disseminates national clinical guidelines containing recommendations for clinicians. www.sign. ac.uk/

Systematic reviews

The Cochrane Library produces and disseminates systematic reviews of healthcare interventions. www.cochrane.org/index.htm

Clinical Evidence produced by the BMJ, is a compendium of evidence for effective healthcare organised for easy reference (available to NHS staff in Scotland and Wales and some other healthcare systems worldwide). www.clinicalevidence.org

Mind map

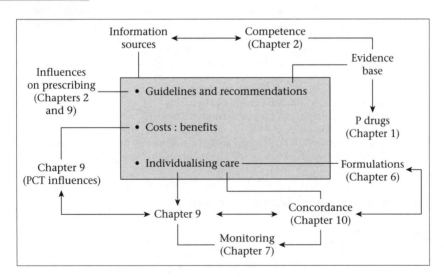

12

Conclusion

Trudy Thomas

I hope that you have enjoyed working through the scenarios in this book and that you have found useful information and advice to apply to and enhance your own prescribing practice. Learning to prescribe is something that you will continue to do throughout your career – it is never something that you can tick off as 'done'. However, the rewards of your continual development in this area of practice will be life-changing for both your patients and yourself.

Index